医学・医療系学生のための

総合医学英語テキスト Step2

English for Medical Purposes, Step 2
JASMEE

日本医学英語教育学会 編
The Japan Society for Medical English Education (JASMEE)

MEDICAL VIEW

English for Medical Purposes, Step 2 (JASMEE)
(ISBN 978–4–7583–0449–8 C3347)

Edited by the Japan Society for Medical English Education (JASMEE)

2017.10.1   1st edition

©MEDICAL VIEW, 2017
Printed and Bound in Japan

Medical View Co., Ltd.
2–30 Ichigaya-hommuracho, Shinjuku-ku, Tokyo 162–0845, Japan
E-mail ed@medicalview.co.jp

刊行にあたって

　文部科学省では「グローバル化に対応した英語教育改革実施計画」のもとに，小・中・高等学校を通じた英語教育全体の抜本的充実を図っている。2014年度から逐次改革を推進し，一貫した学習到達目標を設定することにより，英語によるコミュニケーション能力を確実に養うことを目指している。

　医学教育においてもグローバル化への対応が進んでいる。2017年に改訂された医学教育モデル・コア・カリキュラムのなかでは，「A-7-2）国際医療への貢献」の項で，「患者の文化的背景を尊重し，英語をはじめとした異なる言語に対応することができる」ことが学修目標として掲げられている。

　さて，わが国の医学教育は，世界医学教育連盟（WFME）のグローバルスタンダード評価基準に準拠して進められており，各学校においても国際認証に向けた取り組みが行われている。日本医学英語教育学会では，わが国の医学英語教育がWFMEのグローバルスタンダードに基づくよう，いち早く医学英語教育のガイドラインを制定した（*J Med Eng Educ* 14（3）:130-135, 136-142, 2015）。そして，ガイドラインに基づく理想的な教育が行えるよう，テキストを制作するに至った。このテキストは，医学英語運用における重要な4技能（Vocabulary, Reading, Writing, Communication）それぞれを網羅しており，12回の講義で使用できるように工夫した。すでに，医学部低学年や医療系学生を対象とし，一般的症候をトピックとしたStep 1が刊行されているが，この度，医学部高学年や医師を対象とし，医学的知識が必要な内容をトピックとするStep 2を刊行するに至った。

　このStep 2では「医師国家試験出題基準」に収載されている主要疾患をトピックとして取り上げ，また過去に出題された試験問題も練習問題として取り上げている。医療系大学における教科書として使用できることを前提に，専門的医学的知識をもたない英語教員でも講義が進められるよう，教師用マニュアルも用意されている。また，医師が生涯教育の一環としても利用できるよう，医療画像や臨床現場を再現した状況での英語会話などが用意されている。卒前教育から卒後の生涯教育において本書が広く利用され，わが国における医療人の英語力向上につながることを期待している。

　最後になりましたが，本書の作成に多大な尽力をいただいた，メジカルビュー社の江口潤司氏，石田奈緒美氏に厚く御礼申し上げます。

2017年9月吉日

編著者を代表して

一杉 正仁

日本医学英語教育学会
副理事長・テキスト編集委員会 委員長
滋賀医科大学 社会医学講座

執筆者一覧

■ 編集

日本医学英語教育学会　医学英語テキスト編集委員会

委員長：	一杉　　正仁	滋賀医科大学 社会医学講座（法医学部門）教授
委員：	福沢　　嘉孝	愛知医科大学病院 先制・統合医療包括センター　センター長
	森　　　茂	大分大学医学部 医学英語教育学 教授
	安藤　　千春	獨協医科大学医学部 特任教授
	Clive Langham	日本大学歯学部 教授
	Timothy Minton	慶應義塾大学医学部 英語 教授

■ 執筆（掲載順）

黒住　　和彦	岡山大学大学院医歯薬学総合研究科 脳神経外科 講師
小島 多香子	東京医科大学 国際医学情報学分野 講師
永山　　正雄	国際医療福祉大学医学部 神経内科学 教授
濱西　　和子	北陸学院大学 非常勤講師
高田　　淳	高知大学医学部 医学教育創造・推進室 教授
玉巻　　欣子	神戸薬科大学 英語 准教授
五十嵐 裕章	河北総合病院 副院長・内科部長
服部 しのぶ	藤田保健衛生大学医療科学部 臨床工学科 准教授
福沢　　嘉孝	愛知医科大学病院 先制・統合医療包括センター　センター長
森　　　茂	大分大学医学部 医学英語教育学 教授
入交　　重雄	りんくう総合医療センター 総合内科感染症内科・国際診療科・膠原病内科 部長
川越　　栄子	神戸女学院大学 教授
相見　　良成	滋賀医科大学医学部看護学科 基礎看護学 教授
平野 美津子	元・聖隷クリストファー大学リハビリテーション学部 教授
守屋　　利佳	北里大学医学部 医学教育研究開発センター 准教授
大下　　晴美	大分大学医学部 医学英語教育学 准教授
亀岡　　淳一	東北医科薬科大学医学部 内科学第三（血液・リウマチ科）教授
鈴木　　光代	東京女子医科大学医学部 英語 准教授
青木　　洋介	佐賀大学医学部 国際医療学講座・臨床感染症学分野 教授
芦田　　ルリ	東京慈恵会医科大学 国際交流センター 教授
塩田　　充	川崎医科大学 婦人科腫瘍学教室 教授
松本　　珠希	四天王寺大学教育学部 保健教育コース 教授
一杉　　正仁	滋賀医科大学社会医学講座（法医学部門）教授
安藤　　千春	獨協医科大学医学部 特任教授

■ 編集協力

Christopher Holmes	東京大学医学部 国際交流室 講師

Contents

1. Cerebrovascular disease ······ 黒住和彦，小島多香子　　1

2. Epilepsy ···················· 永山正雄，濱西和子　17

3. Acute myocardial infarction ····· 高田　淳，玉巻欣子　31

4. Inflammatory bowel disease ·· 五十嵐裕章，服部しのぶ　45

5. Cirrhosis of the liver ············· 福沢嘉孝，森　茂　59

6. Rheumatoid arthritis and systemic lupus erythematosus
 ···················· 入交重雄，川越栄子　75

7. Diabetes mellitus ············ 相見良成，平野美津子　89

8. Chronic kidney disease ········· 守屋利佳，大下晴美　103

9. Malignant lymphoma ··········· 亀岡淳一，鈴木光代　115

10. Infective endocarditis ·········· 青木洋介，芦田ルリ　129

11. Uterine fibroid ················ 塩田　充，松本珠希　145

12. Head trauma ················· 一杉正仁，安藤千春　159

 Index ·································· 173

各章のMedical communicationで使用する音声はメジカルビュー社ホームページからダウンロード可能です。ダウンロード方法については，次ページをご参照ください。

本書の使い方

Pre-reading activities

　各章で扱うトピックに関連する質問が示されています。インターネットや学術文献で事前に調べてから授業に臨みましょう。

I. Reading

　Readingは各章のトピックに関連する読み物です。内容を理解するとともに，Comprehension questionsで理解度を確認しましょう。

II. Vocabulary

　Vocabularyには各章のトピックに関連する重要な用語が掲載されています。基本となる用語ばかりですので，すべて覚えるようにしましょう。

　また専門用語に関する解説や医学的知識（Medical Background）についても簡単に解説しています。

III. Medical communication

　各章のMedical communicationで使用する音声データは，メジカルビュー社のホームページからダウンロードできます。〈http://www.medicalview.co.jp/download/〉

　まずテキストを読む前に，会話を聞きながら会話の下線部を埋め，またClinical exercisesに答えてください。

　その後で下線部の正解を確認しながら，会話でよく使われる表現を覚えましょう。

IV. Further Study

　Further Studyでは，さらに理解を深めるための課題が示されています。インターネットや学術文献で調べて，得られた情報を患者さんに説明するときのように平易な英語で説明してみましょう。

■音声ダウンロード方法

①下記URLにアクセスしてください。

　http://www.medicalview.co.jp/download/ISBN978-4-7583-0449-8

②本書の音声再生ページが表示されますので，利用規約に同意の上，ご利用ください。「音声を聴く」ボタンをクリックすると音声が再生されます。ダウンロードする場合はご使用のブラウザのヘルプをご覧ください。

注）お使いのPC端末の種類やブラウザによっては正常に再生・ダウンロードできない場合があります。

　本書の解答集をご希望の方にお分けいたします（ただし，授業の教材として利用されている学生の方は除きます）。ご希望の方は必ず書面（FAX，E-mailも可）にて，氏名・勤務先・送付先住所を明記のうえ，下記へお申し込みください。

　申込先：メジカルビュー社 編集部 医学英語書籍担当者

　　　〒162-0845　東京都新宿区市谷本村町2-30

　　　FAX　0120-77-2062　　E-mail　ed@medicalview.co.jp

日本医学英語教育学会

医学教育のグローバルスタンダードに
対応するための
医学英語教育ガイドライン

日本医学英語教育学会 ガイドライン委員会

【本ガイドラインの構成】

　本ガイドラインにおいては，英語運用能力（proficiency）を下記の4項目に分類している。

(1) Vocabulary

(2) Reading

(3) Writing

(4) Communication

　学習のoutcomeとして，医学部卒業時に全員が習得すべき内容をMinimum requirements，全員が習得する必要はないが，さらなる能力向上のために習得が望ましい内容を Advanced requirementsと定義した。そして前記の4運用能力それぞれに対して，学習目標を大別して具体的に示した。Minimum requirementsは次頁以降に示す通りである。

(*Journal of Medical English Education* 2015; 14(3): 130–135 より引用)

Minimum requirements

(1) Vocabulary

- 身体の部位と機能，医療・健康に関する基本的な専門用語を理解し使うことができる。
- 医学英単語を使い，必要な情報を英語テキストやweb上で検索できる。

［具体的な目安］

〈基本的な英単語（一般用語と専門用語語彙）〉

- 「身体の部位と機能」，「症状，徴候」，「検査，診療行為，診療器具」，「疾患，診断」に関する基本的な専門用語を理解し使うことができる。
  注）基本的な専門用語：医師国家試験出題基準に記載されている医学用語に相当する英語表記。

〈英語表現〉

- 「医療面接」，「身体診察」，「患者への病状説明や指示・指導」「医療情報（カルテ，電子カルテ）記載」，「症例プレゼンテーション」で必要な基本的な英語表現を使うことができる。
- 医学・医療の研究に必要な英単語，英語表現の情報を英語テキストやweb上で検索できる。

(2) Reading

- 医療・健康に必要な基本的な医学英語が理解できる。
- 医学・医療の研究の基礎に必要な医学英語が理解できる。

［具体的な目安］

〈診療〉

- 基本的な身体機能及び疾患の英語表記を理解できる。
- 基本的な症状，徴候の英語表記を理解できる。
- 基本的な診察所見，診療行為，診療器具の英語表記を理解できる。
- 基本疾患（モデル・コア・カリキュラムに収載されている）について英語の資料を読み，内容を理解できる。

〈研究〉

- 英語の文献検索を行い，目的とする英語論文のabstractを読んで理解できる。
- 医学英語論文の基本的な構造を理解できる（abstract, introduction, methods, results, discussion, references）。

(3) Writing

- テクニカル・ライティングができる。
- 医学・医療関連のインフォーマルなコミュニケーション英文が書ける。
- 医学・医療の英文abstractを書ける。

［具体的な目安］

〈テクニカル・ライティング〉

- テクニカル・ライティングの存在を知っている。
- パラグラフ・ライティングができる。
- 一貫性（coherence）の保たれた文章を書ける。
- 明確（clear）かつ簡潔（concise）な文章を書ける。
- 推敲（self-editing）ができる。

〈一般のコミュニケーション英文〉
・基本的な文法（punctuationを含む）を知っている。
・基本的な語彙（医学用語を含む）を知っている。
・応用的な文法・語彙を調べながら運用できる。
・インフォーマル文書（e-mail, etc.）を書ける。
〈医学英語論文（およびそれに準じたレポート）〉
・医学論文に必要な要素を理解している。
・英文abstractを自分で書ける。

(4) Communication

・英語で患者を案内することや良好な関係を築くことができ，基本的な医療面接を行える。
・英語で医学・医療の研究成果の簡単な発表と質疑応答ができる。

　注　Minimum requirementは「国内における外国人患者への対応」を前提とする。

［具体的な目安］
〈診療〉
・聴解力
　・一般的な身体表現，症状を聴き取り，理解できる。
　・専門用語を使用した医療従事者間の会話を聴き取り，理解できる。
・発話力
　・初診患者の受付や院内誘導などの案内ができる。
　・挨拶・患者確認，ならびに基本的な医療面接を行える。
　・患者の診察上必要な説明（体位の変換，指示など）を行える。
〈研究〉
・聴解力
　・（英語を母語としない人たちを対象とした）国際学会発表などのプレゼンテーションの内容をおおむね理解できる。
　・（英語を母語としない人たちを対象とした）グループディスカッションでの議論の内容をおおむね理解できる。
　・医学・医療関連の英語メディアの情報を聴き取りおおむね理解できる。
・発話力
　・簡単なプレゼンテーションができる。
　・グループディスカッションで自分の意見を簡単に述べることができる。
　・簡単な質問に答えることができる。

　なお，Advanced requirementsも含めたガイドラインの詳細については，日本医学英語教育学会ホームページに掲載されているので，参照されたい。

日本医学英語教育学会ホームページ〈https://jasmee.jp〉

1. Cerebrovascular disease

　脳血管障害（cerebrovascular disease）は死因の一つとなる代表的な疾患であり，血管が破れる脳出血と血管が詰まる脳梗塞の2つに分類されます。さらに脳出血は脳内出血とくも膜下出血，脳梗塞は脳血栓症および脳塞栓症に分類されます。高齢化社会や生活習慣病の増加により，患者数は増加していますが，その予防や治療は年々進歩してきています。

Pre-reading activities

Do the following exercise before the class.

1. **What does the term "cerebrovascular disease" mean?**

   ....

2. **What are the main types of cerebrovascular disease?**

   ....

3. **What are the symptoms of cerebrovascular disease?**

   ....

4. **What kind of treatment is given for cerebrovascular disease?**

   ....

5. **How many people have cerebrovascular disease in the United States?**

   ....

I. Reading

Read the following passages, and answer the questions that follow it.

Passage 1

Cerebrovascular disease, sometimes called a brain attack (stroke), occurs when the blood supply to part of the brain is blocked or when a blood vessel in the brain bursts. A stroke can cause lasting brain damage, long-term disability, or death.

brain attack 脳発作

burst 破裂する

Epidemiology of cerebrovascular disease

Stroke is the fifth leading cause of death in the United States, killing more than 130,000 Americans each year—that's 1 of every 20 deaths.

The 2 main types of stroke are ischemic stroke and hemorrhagic stroke (**Figure 1**).

ischemic stroke 虚血性脳卒中

Ischemic stroke

An ischemic stroke occurs when blood clots or other particles block the blood vessels to the brain. Plaque deposits can also cause blockages by building up in the blood vessels. An ischemic stroke can be either a thrombotic, embolic or transient ischemic attack.

plaque プラーク

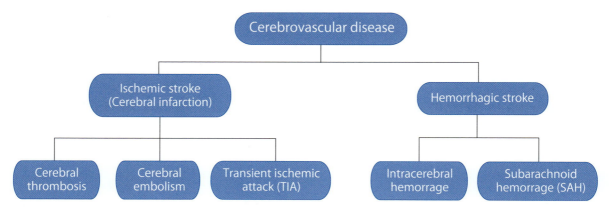

Figure 1.   Classification of cerebrovascular disease.

• Cerebral thrombosis

Cerebral thrombosis refers to a thrombus (blood clot) that develops at the clogged[1] part of the vessel.

thrombus 血栓

clogged 詰まった

• Cerebral embolism

A cerebral embolism is a blood clot that forms at another location in the heart, and large arteries of the upper chest and neck becomes loose and travels through blood vessels of the brain. One of the main causes of embolism is an irregular heartbeat (e.g. atrial fibrillation).

• Transient ischemic attack (TIA)

TIA is a short episode of stroke-like symptoms that appear suddenly and last for several minutes to a few hours. More than half of all strokes are preceded by TIAs.

Symptoms include
- headache
- dizziness or confusion
- weakness in one side of the body
- sudden, severe numbness[2] in any part of the body
- visual disturbance
- walking difficulty
- slurred speech or inability to speak

confusion 錯乱

Any of these symptoms can appear suddenly. Symptoms may stay the same or gradually become worse, over a few hours or days.

Computed tomography (CT) and magnetic resonance imaging (MRI) are useful for diagnosis. Usually the CT scan is done first. If the CT scan does not show any sign of bleeding, it can be suspected that a blocked artery from a blood clot is

1. Cerebrovascular disease　3

causing the stroke. An MRI is performed when it is necessary to confirm brain injury changes consistent with a new ischemic stroke. Diffusion weighted imaging (DWI) is used for early identification of ischemic strokes. Fluid-attenuated inversion recovery imaging (FLAIR) can detect the ischemic area six to twelve hours after initial onset (**Figure 2**).

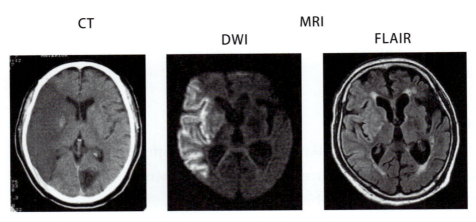

Figure 2.　Radiological images in cerebral ischemia.

Acute-phase treatment is given in the form of intravenous injection of tissue plasminogen activator (tPA). For longer term treatment of thrombotic strokes, an anti-platelet agent is prescribed. For embolic strokes, an oral anti-coagulant drug, such as warfarin, or a novel oral anti-coagulant drug is prescribed.

Recently, a procedure called mechanical thrombectomy has become a new modality of treatment for acute ischemic stroke. This treatment is initiated within six hours of acute stroke symptom onset. To remove the blood clot that is blocking an artery in the brain, a catheter is threaded through an artery in the groin to the site of the blood clot. The stent opens and grabs the clot, allowing doctors to trap and remove the clot and restore blood flow.

novel 新しい

mechanical thrombectomy 機械的血栓除去術

groin 鼠径部

Comprehension questions 1

1. **What is the pathogenesis of an ischemic stroke?**

   ....

2. **Give a brief description of the 3 types of ischemic stroke.**

   ....

3. **How is an ischemic stroke diagnosed?**

   ....

Passage 2

Hemorrhagic stroke

A hemorrhagic stroke occurs when a blood vessel bursts in the brain. Blood builds up and damages the surrounding brain tissue. There are 2 kinds of hemorrhagic stroke: intracerebral hemorrhage and subarachnoid hemorrhage.

intracerebral hemorrhage 脳内出血

• Intracerebral hemorrhage

Intracerebral hemorrhage is the most common type of hemorrhagic stroke. It occurs when an artery in the brain bursts, flooding the surrounding tissue with blood. Some factors that increase the risk of this kind of hemorrhage are high blood pressure (hypertension), heavy alcohol intake, and advanced age. Less common causes of intracerebral hemorrhage include trauma, infections, tumors, blood clotting deficiencies, and abnormalities in the blood vessels (such as arteriovenous malformations).

blood clotting deficiency 血液凝固因子欠乏

malformation 奇形

Symptoms include
• paralysis or numbness in any part of the body
• speech disturbance

1. Cerebrovascular disease 5

- vomiting
- difficulty walking
- stupor
- coma

Symptoms tend to appear without warning, but they can develop gradually.

CT or MRI scan can be useful for imaging diagnosis. For hemorrhagic strokes, CT scans are the fastest and most effective test of imaging.

Medication to control high blood pressure and reduce brain swelling that follows a stroke is prescribed. In some cases, surgery is necessary to remove a large portion of the clot after a hemorrhage.

• Subarachnoid hemorrhage (SAH)

Subarachnoid hemorrhage is a less common type of hemorrhagic stroke. It refers to bleeding into the subarachnoid space, which is between the pial and arachnoid membranes.

Symptoms include
- a very severe headache that starts suddenly
- nausea and vomiting
- stiff neck
- dizziness
- confusion
- loss of consciousness

For hemorrhagic strokes, CT scans are the fastest and most effective imaging test of the brain (**Figure 3**). MRI angiography can provide information about the blood flow to the brain. If a subarachnoid hemorrhage is not detected with image studies, a lumbar puncture will be performed. This mainly

stupor 昏迷

pial 軟膜
arachnoid くも膜

lumbar puncture
腰椎穿刺

occurs in ruptured cerebral aneurysms.

    Surgery is often performed to place a metal clip at the neck of an aneurysm. Some procedures are less invasive. A catheter is used to be inserted into a major artery of the leg or arm. The catheter is guided to the aneurysm where it places a device, such as a coil, to prevent rupture.

less invasive
低侵襲な

(Adapted from: https://www.cdc.gov/stroke/about.htm; http://www.strokeassociation.org/STROKEORG/AboutStroke/TypesofStroke/IschemicClots/; https://www.drugs.com/health-guide/hemorrhagic-stroke.html)

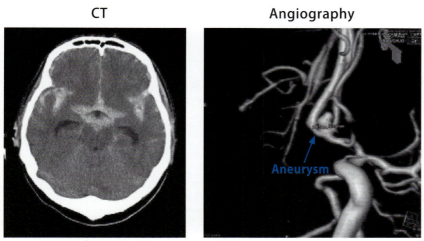

Figure 3.　Radiological images in SAH.

Comprehension questions 2

1. What is the pathogenesis of a hemorrhagic stroke?

2. What is the difference between an intracerebral hemorrhage and a subarachnoid hemorrhage?

3. What are the risk factors for an intracerebral hemorrhage?

II. Vocabulary

☐ acute thrombectomy	急性期血栓除去療法
☐ aneurysm	動脈瘤
☐ angiography	血管撮影〔法〕
☐ anti-coagulant drug	抗凝固薬
☐ anti-platelet drug	抗血小板薬
☐ atherosclerosis	動脈硬化〔症〕
☐ atherosclerotic plaque	アテローム性動脈硬化性プラーク
☐ atrial fibrillation	心房細動
☐ basilar artery	脳底動脈
☐ computed tomography, computerized axial tomography, CAT scan	コンピュータ連動断層撮影〔法〕，CTスキャン《海外ではCTではなくCATとよばれることも多い》
☐ clipping	クリッピング術
☐ cerebrovascular disease	脳血管障害
☐ cerebral infarction	脳梗塞
☐ cerebral thrombosis	脳血栓症
☐ coil embolization	コイル塞栓術
☐ diffusion weighted image (DWI)	拡散強調画像
☐ embolism	塞栓症
☐ embolus	塞栓
☐ endovascular surgery	血管内治療
☐ fluid-attenuated inversion recovery (FLAIR)	フレアー法
☐ hyperlipidemia	高脂血症
☐ intensive therapy	集中治療
☐ language therapy	言語療法
☐ middle cerebral artery	中大脳動脈
☐ occupational therapy (OT)	作業療法

☐ physical therapy (PT)	理学療法
☐ posterior cerebral artery	後大脳動脈
☐ posterior communicating artery	後交通動脈
☐ prognosis	予後
☐ subarachnoid hemorrhage (SAH)	くも膜下出血
☐ single photon emission computed tomography (SPECT)	スペクト
☐ thrombolytic therapy	血栓溶解療法
☐ thrombosis	血栓症
☐ thrombus	血栓
☐ tissue-type plasminogen activator (t-PA, tPA)	組織プラスミノーゲン・アクチベータ
☐ transient ischemic attack (TIA)	一過性脳虚血発作
☐ vertebral artery	椎骨動脈

III. Medical communication

Listen to the recording of the following case report and fill in the blanks. Then do the exercises that follow.

Case report

A ____-year-old man was found lying _____, and was immediately _____ to our hospital. He had been taking medication for _____ for 10 years, and was receiving an angiotensin receptor blocker. He had no _____ and he did not smoke.

On _____, he was unconscious (Glasgow Coma Scale E1V1M2), and his blood pressure was 210/95 mmHg; his heart rate was 95/min and regular, his respiratory rate was 18 /min, and his body temperature was 37.2°C. His right _____ was 4.0 mm in diameter, the left pupil was 5.0 mm, and the pupillary light _____ was _____.

Laboratory data on admission showed a prothrombin time (PT) of 9.5 seconds, and a PT/international normalized _____ (INR) of 0.81.

A CT scan of the brain _____ hematomas in the right lateral putamen. The size of the _____ was 7×3×4 cm. CT also indicated the _____ of blood in the ventricles (Figure 4). As the hematomas were large and the patient's _____ condition was _____, surgery was performed.

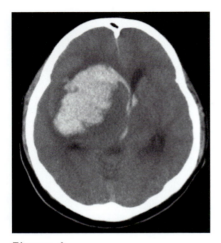

Figure 4.

Clinical exercises

1. **What was the cause of the patient's loss of consciousness?**

   a   Hypoglycemia

   b   Intracranial hemorrhage

   c   Hypoxic encephalopathy

   d   Encephalitis

   e   Hepatic encephalopathy

2. **Which of the following examinations would be useful for diagnostic purposes? Choose two.**

   a   Abdominal echography

   b   Head CT

   c   Head MRI

   d   Neuroendoscopy

   e   Brain X-ray

3. **Which of the following medications would be appropriate?**

   a   Anti-coagulant

   b   Anti-platelet agent

   c   Anti-hypertensive drug

   d   Chemotherapeutic agent

   e   Hypoglycemic agent

Check your answers.

Case report

A **48**-year-old man was found lying **unconscious**, and was immediately **admitted**[3] to our hospital. He had been taking medication for **hypertension** for 10 years, and was receiving an angiotensin receptor blocker. He had no **allergies** and he did not smoke.

On **admission**, he was unconscious (Glasgow Coma Scale E1V1M2), and his blood pressure was 210/95 mmHg; his heart rate was 95/min and regular, his respiratory rate was 18 /min, and his body temperature was 37.2°C. His right **pupil** was 4.0 mm in diameter, the left pupil was 5.0 mm, and the pupillary light **reflex** was **sluggish**.[4]

Laboratory data on admission showed a prothrombin time (PT) of 9.5 seconds, and a PT/international normalized **ratio** (INR) of 0.81.

A CT scan of the brain **revealed** hematomas in the right lateral putamen. The size of the **hemorrhage** was 7×3×4 cm. CT also indicated the **presence** of blood in the ventricles (Figure 4). As the hematomas were large and the patient's **neurological** condition was **severe**, surgery was performed.

angiotensin receptor blocker アンジオテンシン受容体遮断薬

Glasgow Coma Scale グラスゴー・コーマ・スケール

pupil 瞳孔

light reflex 対光反射
sluggish 鈍い

right lateral putamen 右外側被殻

hematoma 血腫

> **Note how the following common terms and phrases are used in case reports.**

❶ clogged

「詰まった」の意味。

Fat can cause your arteries **to clog up**. (脂肪が動脈を詰まらせることがある。)

Clogged arteries can lead to a heart attack or stroke.

(動脈が詰まると心臓発作や脳卒中につながることがある。)

他にも

clogged-up nose: 詰まった鼻

My nose is **clogged up**, so I'm finding it difficult to sleep.
(鼻が詰まっているので寝つきが悪い。)

clogged pores: 詰まった毛穴

Clogged pores can give you acne.
(毛穴が詰まるとニキビになることがある。)

❷ numbness

「しびれ，無感覚」の意味。numbは他にも次のような使い方をする。

My fingers were so cold that they **felt numb.**

My leg **felt numb**. (feel numb しびれているように感じる)

My leg **went numb**. (go numb しびれる，しびれさせる)

I had a **numb feeling** in my leg. (numb feeling しびれた感覚)

One of the symptoms of stroke is **numbness** in one side of the body.

(脳卒中の症状の一つは身体の片側のしびれである。)

❸ He was admitted

admitは一般的には「入ることを認められる」という意味。

例えば，He **was admitted** to X University in 2014. (彼は2014年にx大学に入学を許可された。)

しかし，症例報告や医学論文などで使用する場合は「入院する」という意味で使われる。

He was **admitted** because of a broken leg. (彼は骨折のため入院した。)

❹ sluggish

sluggishは「動きが鈍い，のろい，不活発」などの意味がある。ちなみにslugとは英語でナメクジの意味。

She felt tired and **sluggish**. (彼女は疲れて体がだるい感じがした。)

1. Cerebrovascular disease   13

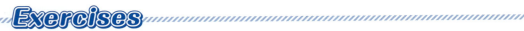

1. **Fill in the blanks to complete the following doctor-patient interview.**

   Doctor: _____?

   Patient: Yes, I've been taking an angiotensin receptor blocker for my high blood pressure.

   Doctor: _____?

   Patient: Oh, for about 10 years now.

   Doctor: Are you allergic to anything?

   Patient: _____, not that I know of.

   Doctor: _____?

   Patient: No, I've never smoked in my life.

2. **How would you say the following in English?**

   A. 症状は何の前触れもなく現れることが多い。

   _____

   B. CT画像所見で腫瘍が認められた。

   _____

IV. Further Study

Search for information about therapies for cerebrovascular disease, including those under investigation, through the Internet and academic papers. Also briefly explain the obtained information in simple English, the way you would do when talking to a patient.

A. Medication

B. Surgery

C. Nutritional therapy

D. Novel approaches (endovascular surgery, regenerative medicine)

COLUMN

英文ライティングのルール ❶ 英文を書くときは欧文フォントを使う

　日本語は，漢字・ひらがな・カタカナが
すべて同じサイズに収まるように作られ
ていて，これを「全角文字」と称します。
一方，欧文は文字によって幅や高さが異な
り，これを「半角文字」と称しています。
したがって同じアルファベットでも全角
と半角では下記のように違いがあります。

● 全角　　a b c d e f g h i j k l m n
　　　　　o p q r s t u v w x z

● 半角　　abcdefghijklmnopqrstuvwxyz

　全角文字だと前後にスペースが入って
いるように見えますので，英文は半角文字
を使わなくてはなりません。

　また日本語フォントでも半角文字でア
ルファベットを表示することはできます
が，欧文フォントを使った方が，英文とし
ての仕上がりはきれいですし，文字によっ
ては細かい違いもあります。また将来，英
語論文を投稿する際には，海外のPCでは
日本語フォントは表示できないので，無用
のトラブルを招く元にもなります。英文を
書くときは，欧文専用フォント（Timesや
Helveticaなど）を使うようにしましょう。

2. Epilepsy

　てんかん（epilepsy）とは，脳の慢性疾患であって，大脳ニューロンの過剰な発射（てんかん放電）に由来する反復性の発作（てんかん発作epileptic seizure）をきたす神経疾患あるいは症状です。

　広義には救急患者の40〜60％は神経救急・集中治療を必要とします。重症患者の20％以上は神経系合併症を有し，最も多いのはてんかん発作（痙攣性，非痙攣性）です。発作が5分以上持続する場合，てんかん重積状態（status epilepticus）とよびます。近年，高頻度，重症で多彩な症状を示す非痙攣性てんかん重積状態が注目されています。

Pre-reading activities

Do the following exercise before the class.

1. **What is an epileptic seizure?**

2. **What is epilepsy? How is it different from an epileptic seizure?**

3. **What are the symptoms of an epileptic seizure?**

4. **Do epileptic seizures always involve convulsions?**

5. **What is status epilepticus?**

6. **How can epileptic seizures be prevented?**

I. Reading

Read the following passage, and answer the questions that follow it.

What are epileptic seizures?

Epileptic seizures are episodes of vigorous uncontrolled movements of varying duration, including convulsions and shaking. A seizure occurs when there is a sudden burst of intense electrical activity in the brain causing a temporary disruption to the way the brain normally works.

episode 発作
vigorous 強い, 活発な

disruption 中断, 途絶

What is epilepsy?

Epilepsy is a functional disorder that affects the brain and is characterized by epileptic seizures. In patients with epilepsy, seizures recur without any immediate underlying cause.[1] Isolated seizures due to a specific cause such as meningitis and poisoning are not considered as epilepsy. Epilepsy can start at any age and is often a life-long condition. If a seizure lasts longer than 5 minutes, or if there are more than two seizures an hour without a return to normal levels of consciousness between them, this is called status epilepticus, a critical condition which needs emergency intensive care. Status epilepticus is usually categorized as convulsive status epilepticus (CSE) or nonconvulsive status epilepticus (NCSE).

underlying cause
根本 (根底にある) 原因, 遠因
isolated seizure
孤立発作
life-long condition
一生涯継続する状態

Manifestations

Convulsive seizures can be tonic or clonic. In addition to convulsive seizures, there are many other types of seizure, depending on the part of the brain affected. Some people may remain alert, while others may lose awareness and have unusual sensations, feelings, movements or behaviors. If epileptic seizures are nonconvulsive, they are frequently missed, even by physicians. Manifestations of NCSE now include not only classical features, such as staring, repetitive blinking, chewing, swallowing and automatism, but also coma, prolonged apnea, cardiac arrest, dementia, and higher brain dysfunction.

prolonged apnea
遷延性無呼吸

Prevalence

Epilepsy is one of the most common and critical neurological conditions in the world. In 2015, 39 million people were affected worldwide. NCSE is more frequently observed than CSE. If symptomatic epilepsy is included, prevalence is much higher.

Causes

The causes of most cases of epilepsy are unknown. However, symptomatic epilepsy is defined as epileptic seizures resulting from acquired or genetic causes, including traumatic brain injuries, strokes, brain tumors, infections of the central nervous system (e.g. meningitis, encephalitis, and brain abscess), and acute encephalopathy (including post-hypoxic and post-ischemic encephalopathy, and acute metabolic encephalopathy); the seizures of symptomatic epilepsy can also be the result of side effects of medication, complications of diagnostic and therapeutic procedures, intoxication of the nervous system, birth defects, and genetic mutations. Symptomatic epilepsy develops through a process known as epileptogenesis.

encephalitis 脳炎

encephalopathy
脳症
post-hypoxic
低酸素後の
post-ischemic
虚血後の

Diagnosis

A detailed medical interview focusing on seizures and a physical examination are crucial for a diagnosis, that rules out[2] other conditions that might cause similar symptoms. Differential diagnoses include syncope due to various causes, transient ischemic attack, transient neurological attack, non-epileptic seizures, and factitious diseases. Diagnostic work-up[3] includes imaging studies such as blood tests and electroencephalography

crucial 重要な
rule out 除外する

(EEG). However, a normal test result does not rule out the possibility of epileptic seizures, and an abnormal result does not confirm a diagnosis of epileptic seizures. Continuous EEG video monitoring is critically important, especially for diagnosing NCSE.

Management and prevention

Seizures can be controlled with antiepileptic drugs in about 70% of cases. However, status epilepticus is often refractory to initial medications. In cases where seizures do not respond to medication, surgery, vagus nerve stimulation, or a ketogenic diet are considered. Epilepsy and epileptic seizures that occur as a result of other conditions are, of course, preventable if the underlying conditions are resolved. It is also very important to avoid seizure triggers, which include sleep deficit, overwork, excessive alcohol consumption, photic stimuli, and hyperventilation.

initial 最初の
ketogenic diet
ケトン食《「脂肪が多く炭水化物が少ない食事を摂れば絶食と同等の効果が得られる」という考えのもとに，1920年代に米国のMayo Clinicで発案された》

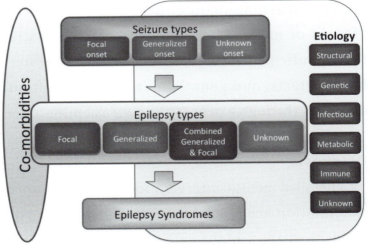

Figure 1. New classification of epilepsy.

2017年3月，International League Against Epilepsy（ILAE）は新しいてんかんの分類を発表した。従来の「部分発作／全般発作」「特発性／全般性」の2軸による4分類法で区分できない疾患概念が指摘されていたため，これに対応できるように「発作分類（seizure types）」「病因（etiology）」「併存疾患（comorbidity）」「てんかん症候群（epilepsy syndrome）」の4軸で分類することを提案している。
（http：//www.ilae.org/Visitors/Centre/Definition_Class.cfm）

Comprehension questions

1. What is nonconvulsive status epilepticus?

   ....

   ....

2. How are epilepsy and epileptic seizures diagnosed?

   ....

   ....

3. List some epileptic seizure triggers.

   ....

   ....

Decide if the following statement is true (T) or false (F) according to the passage.

1. _____ Even for physicians, it is hard to diagnose nonconvulsive status epilepticus.

2. _____ Infections of the central nervous system such as meningitis and encephalitis are types of epilepsy.

3. _____ Status epilepticus is a critical condition requiring immediate emergency intensive care.

4. _____ Nonconvulsive status epilepticus is more frequently observed than convulsive status epilepticus.

5. _____ Initial medications often fail to control status epilepticus.

2. Epilepsy 21

II. Vocabulary

☐ acquired	後天的な（cf. innate）
☐ acute encephalopathy	急性脳症
☐ acute metabolic encephalopathy	急性代謝性脳症
☐ antiepileptic	抗てんかん薬
☐ apnea	無呼吸
☐ automatism	自動症
☐ awareness	認識，自覚
☐ birth defect	先天性欠損
☐ brain abscess	脳膿瘍
☐ coma	昏睡状態
☐ continuous EEG video monitoring	持続ビデオ脳波モニタリング
☐ convulsion	痙攣，発作
☐ convulsive status epilepticus (CSE)	痙攣性てんかん重積状態
☐ cortex	皮質
☐ critical condition	重篤な状態
☐ diagnostic and therapeutic procedures	診断治療手技
☐ electroencephalography (EEG)	脳波検査
☐ emergency intensive care	救急・集中治療
☐ epilepsy	てんかん
☐ epileptic seizure	てんかん発作
☐ epileptogenesis	てんかん原性
☐ factitious disease	虚偽性障害
☐ genetic mutation	遺伝子突然変異
☐ higher brain dysfunction	高次脳機能障害
☐ higher brain function	高次脳機能
☐ hyperventilation	過換気

☐ imaging study	画像診断	
☐ intoxication	中毒	
☐ manifestation	〔症状の〕発現	
☐ neurological condition	神経学的状態（疾患）	
☐ neuron	神経細胞	
☐ nonconvulsive seizure	非痙攣性発作	
☐ nonconvulsive status epilepticus (NCSE)	非痙攣性てんかん重積状態	
☐ non-epileptic seizure	非てんかん性発作	
☐ photic stimulus, [pl.]— stimuli	光刺激	
☐ post-hypoxic and post-ischemic encephalopathy	低酸素後・虚血後脳症	
☐ prevalence	有病率	
☐ prevention	予防	
☐ refractory	難治性の	
☐ repetitive blinking	反復性の瞬目	
☐ seizure	発作	
☐ side effect	〔薬などの〕副作用	
☐ sleep deficit	睡眠不足	
☐ staring	凝視	
☐ status epilepticus	てんかん重積状態	
☐ symptomatic epilepsy	症候性てんかん	
☐ tonic-clonic seizure	強直性間代性発作	
☐ transient neurological attack (TNA)	一過性神経発作	
☐ traumatic brain injury	外傷性脳損傷	
☐ trigger	引き金，誘因	
☐ underlying condition	基礎疾患	
☐ vagus nerve	迷走神経	

Medical Background

疾患のポイント

- てんかん重積状態は，Neurocritical Care Societyにより「臨床的あるいは電気的てんかん活動が少なくとも5分以上続く場合，またはてんかん活動が回復なく反復し5分以上続く場合」と定義されている。
- てんかん重積状態は，痙攣性重積状態（convulsive status epilepticus, CSE）と非痙攣性てんかん重積状態（nonconvulsive status epilepticus, NCSE）に分けられる。
- 抗てんかん薬2剤による適切な初期治療を行ってもてんかん発作が終息しない場合を，難治性てんかん重積状態（refractory status epilepticus, RSE）とよぶ。
- NCSEとは，非痙攣性てんかん発作が持続あるいは反復する重篤な状態である。主に複雑部分発作または単純部分発作が重積する状態で，急性あるいは慢性に新たな表現型を呈するてんかんの一状態像である。
- NCSEの症状は，痙攣発作を呈することなく，凝視，反復性の瞬目・咀嚼・嚥下運動，自動症を呈するほか，昏睡状態，過換気後遷延性無呼吸発作，心静止，呼吸停止による突然死，認知症，さまざまな高次脳機能障害を呈する。

てんかん特性

　てんかん特性の一つは発作が間欠的に反復して出現することであり，熱性痙攣のような散発性のisolated seizure（孤立発作），子癇などのような特定の期間のみに出現するoccasional seizure（機会発作）は，通常は"てんかん"から除外される。しかし，「発作頻度の少ないてんかん発作」（稀発てんかん；oligoepilepsy）とよばれているものが存在し，その診断は臨床上困難であることが多く，また上記てんかんの定義に対して問題を提起しやすい。

（1990　順天堂医学会）

III. Medical communication

Listen to the recording of the following case report and fill in the blanks. Then do the exercises that follow.

Case report

A _____-year-old Japanese male weighing _____ kg, an _____ with a past history of bronchial _____, had had _____ attacks of _____ epileptic seizures. He was referred to the outpatient clinic of the Department of Neurology and emergently _____ to a university hospital.

A _____ medical interview with his family and a physical examination were performed. The patient had a history of _____-_____ seizures and _____ seizures; such seizures had occurred _____ the day before admission. In addition to his epileptic seizures, manifestations included _____ level disturbance (Glasgow Coma Scale E3V3M5), alteration of consciousness, nystagmus of both eyes, and _____ of face and _____.

The attending physician began a _____ work-up which included head CT and MR imaging, electroencephalography (EEG), blood tests for liver function such as AST, ALT, ALP and ammonia, and blood concentration of _____, as well as continuous EEG video monitoring. The work-up disclosed uncompensated liver cirrhosis and hepatic failure, as well as an elevated blood concentration of his medication for bronchial asthma.

With a _____ of mixed convulsive status epilepticus (CSE) and nonconvulsive status epilepticus (NCSE), he was admitted to the Neurological Intensive Care Unit (Neuro-ICU). Intravenous antiepileptic medications were _____ but failed to alleviate his seizures. He was finally sedated with propofol and remifentanil _____ and intubated to secure his airway.

2. Epilepsy   25

Check your answers.

Case report

A **50**-year-old Japanese male weighing **55** kg, an **alcoholic** with a past history of bronchial **asthma**, had had **recurrent** attacks of **convulsive** epileptic seizures. He was referred to the outpatient clinic of the Department of Neurology and emergently admitted to a university hospital.

A **detailed** medical interview with his family and a physical examination were performed. The patient had a history of **tonic**-**clonic** seizures and **nonconvulsive** seizures; such seizures had occurred **repeatedly** the day before admission. In addition to his epileptic seizures, manifestations included **consciousness** level disturbance (Glasgow Coma Scale ❹ E3V3M5), alteration of consciousness, nystagmus of both eyes, and **twitching** of face and **extremities.**

The attending physician began a **diagnostic** work-up which included head CT and MR imaging, electroencephalography (EEG), blood tests for liver function such as AST, ALT, ALP and ammonia, and blood concentration of **antiepileptics**, as well as continuous EEG video monitoring. The work-up disclosed uncompensated liver cirrhosis and hepatic failure, as well as an elevated blood concentration of his medication for bronchial asthma.

With a **diagnosis** of mixed convulsive status epilepticus (CSE) and nonconvulsive status epilepticus (NCSE), he was admitted to the Neurological Intensive Care Unit (Neuro-ICU). Intravenous antiepileptic medications were **administered** but failed to alleviate his seizures. He was finally sedated with propofol and remifentanil **infusions** and intubated to secure his airway. ❺

---

bronchial asthma
気管支喘息
recurrent attack
再発

be referred to
紹介される

alteration 変化

nystagmus 眼振
twitching
ぴくぴく動く

blood
concentration
血中濃度

disclosed
明らかになる，露呈する
hepatic failure
肝不全

intravenous
静脈内の，静脈注射の
点滴による
alleviate 緩和する
anesthetized
麻酔する
propofol
プロポフォール《麻酔薬》

Note how the following common phrases are used in case reports.

❶ underlying cause（根本的原因，遠因）

Histopathology confirmed that the most common **underlying cause** of small bowel obstruction was tuberculosis.（組織病理検査によって，小腸閉塞の最も多い遠因は結核であることが明らかになった。）

❷ rule out（除外する）

鑑別診断の際に，類似した症状から所見に該当しない疾患を排除していく診断方法。

❸ diagnostic work-up（診断ワークアップ）

血液検査やX線撮影など，診断に必要な一連の検査やデータを集めて診断を行うこと。

❹ Glasgow Coma Scale（GCS, グラスゴー・コーマ・スケール）

1974年に英国のグラスゴー大学が発表した意識障害の分類で，現在世界的に広く使用されている評価分類スケール。日本では主に脳神経外科領域で用いられることが多い。開眼・言語・運動の3分野に分けて記録し，意識状態を簡潔かつ的確に記録できる。

❺ He was finally sedated with propofol and remifentanil infusions and intubated to secure his airway.

（彼は最終的にプロポフォールとレミフェンタニルの点滴で鎮静され，挿管により気道を確保された。）

sedateは「（鎮静薬で）落ち着かせる」の意味。propofolは全身麻酔や鎮静に用いられる。remifentanilは超短時間作用性の合成麻薬で全身麻酔に用いられる。infusionは「（静脈への）点滴」，intubateは「挿管する」（気管などにチューブを挿入すること）。

* revive, resuscitate（蘇生する）

He almost died, but artificial respiration was performed to **resuscitate** him.
（彼は死にかけたが，人工呼吸で蘇生した。）

Exercises

- **How will you examine the patient transported by ambulance? Write down the procedure of emergency care in English.**

身体診察

神経学的診察

脈をとる

血圧を測る

血液検査を行う

意識はあるか

震えや痙攣があるか

言葉への反応があるか

四肢の動き，麻痺

凝視

光刺激

瞬目反射

咀嚼

嚥下

自動症

昏睡状態

無呼吸

過換気

認知症／認知障害

脳波

薬物投与

蘇生する*

てんかん発作か，他の脳障害からの発作なのか

IV. Further Study

Search for information about the significance of continuous EEG monitoring in the diagnosis of status epilepticus through the Internet and academic papers. Also briefly explain the obtained information in simple English, the way you would do when talking to a patient.

A. What is continuous electroencephalographic monitoring?

B. To what conditions can the continuous electroencephalographic monitoring be adapted?

C. Speaking practice: Let's present the case report on p.26 in the class.

2. Epilepsy   29

COLUMN

英文ライティングのルール ❷　全角と半角で違う特殊記号

英文ライティングのルール❶（p.16）で説明したように，全角と半角では同じ文字でも違いがあります。特に特殊記号ではその違いが多く，英文としては間違いになってしまうこともあります。例えば，コロンは日本語の全角（：）では前後に空きがありますが，欧文の半角（:）では文字自体に空きはなく，後ろだけにスペースを入れる（: ）のがルールです。そのため，英文の中で全角のコロンを使ってしまうと，誤りになってしまいます。

　全角と半角での主な違いには下記のようなものがあります。

全角	半角	
：	:	高さや前後の空きが違う
（　）	( )	
" "	" "	
' '	' '	
≦	≤	形が違う
℃	℃	欧文では°とCを組み合わせる

　半角の特殊記号はWindowsではAltキーを押しながら4桁の数字を入力して出すことができます。またMacintoshではOptionキーとの組合せで入力できます。

3. Acute myocardial infarction

　急性心筋梗塞（acute myocardial infarction, AMI）は発症時に胸痛を主訴とする疾患で，主に冠状動脈の動脈硬化性病変によって引き起こされます。急性期死亡を防ぐために，発症初期に専門医療機関への早期受診と迅速な初期治療が必要とされる疾患です。近年，その治療の進歩は著しく，従来からの薬物療法に加えて，カテーテル治療（catheter intervention）の飛躍的な向上により，急性期死亡率は顕著に改善しました。

Pre-reading activities

Do the following exercise before the class.

1. **What does the term "ischemia" mean?**

2. **What does the term "infarction" mean?**

3. **What are coronary arteries? Describe their anatomy and function.**

4. **What are the symptoms of acute myocardial infarction?**

5. **Who are likely to be affected by myocardial infarction?**

6. **What treatments are used for acute myocardial infarction?**

I. Reading

Read the following passages and answer the questions that follow them.

Passage 1

Acute myocardial infarction (AMI) is classified within the spectrum of acute coronary syndrome (ACS). ACS includes AMI, unstable angina and cardiac sudden death. Ischemic heart disease, including AMI, is induced by the stenosis of coronary arteries due to atherosclerotic lesions in these vessels. In general, chest pain occurs when the cross-sectional area of a vessel is reduced by 70%–80%. Rupture of the fibrous cap which covers the lipid core in atheroma is an important causal factor of AMI. Subsequent rapid thrombus formation blocks coronary arteries completely.

Risk factors of AMI

The well-known traditional risk factors of atherosclerotic lesions include dyslipidemia (high low-density lipoprotein (LDL), low high-density lipoprotein (HDL) and high triglyceride), diabetes, hypertension, smoking, family history of ischemic heart disease, and mental stress. Evidence of additional risk factors such as C-reactive protein, fibrinogen, lipoprotein(a), and homocysteine have also been reported. Recently, combined risk factors such as metabolic syndrome or chronic kidney disease have been reported with keen interest.

Epidemiology of AMI

According to a report from the Japanese Ministry of Health, Labour and Welfare, there were 196,000 annual cardiovascular deaths in 2014. Among these, 39,000 deaths were attributed to AMI and 35,000 were due to ischemic heart diseases other than AMI. The male-to-female ratio for fatal AMI was 1.26. Despite the male dominancy of atherosclerotic disease, considerable numbers of women died of AMI. Domestic and international

---

spectrum スペクトル《連続する範囲, 概念》

stenosis 狭窄

atherosclerotic lesion アテローム（粥状）硬化性病変

cross-sectional area 断面積

lipoprotein リポ蛋白

triglyceride 中性脂肪

C-reactive protein C反応性蛋白

fibrinogen フィブリノーゲン《血液凝固因子の一つ》

homocysteine ホモシステイン《血中に存在するアミノ酸の一種》

registration studies of AMI showed that the mean age at the onset of AMI was approximately 7 to 8 years higher in women than that in men.

registration study
登録調査
mean 平均〔値〕

Comprehension questions 1

1. What is the mechanism of ischemic heart disease?

   ....

   ....

2. What are the traditional risk factors of atherosclerosis?

   ....

   ....

3. How many patients died of AMI every year?

   ....

Passage 2

Complications of AMI

Because of improvements in the treatment for early-stage AMI, the survival rate of AMI has drastically improved. However, there are still several severe complications which require careful management. Causes of unexpected sudden deaths in early-stage AMI are mainly lethal ventricular arrhythmias (ventricular tachycardia and ventricular fibrillation). Other arrhythmias such as atrial fibrillation or atrio-ventricular block are also important but they are transient. In cases of extensive myocardial infarction, cardiogenic shock due to acute circulatory failure and congestive heart failure with pulmonary edema are possible. Mechanical complications such as papillary muscle rupture, ventricular septal perforation and ventricular free wall rupture with cardiac tamponade are severe complications and can be fatal without prompt and adequate treatments such as surgical intervention.

Treatment of AMI

Any delay in seeking treatment for AMI significantly influences clinical course and prognosis. Many factors such as old age, sex (women), impaired cognitive function, living alone and low education level are reported to be associated with this delay. It is important that patients visit a tertiary medical center by ambulance without significant delay after the onset of symptoms. Patients who recognize that their chest symptoms are related to serious heart problems decide to visit hospital sooner than those who do not. Therefore education programs for the general public and patients are crucial. Establishing safe and prompt systems for patient transport is also necessary. After admission, oxygen supply is started under bed rest, and in cases of severe chest pain, a combination of nitrate and analgesics such as morphine is effective. Anti-platelet agents such as Aspirin quickly prevent thrombus formation. Nitrate and other vasodilators are useful for improving myocardial ischemia and hemodynamic impairment. For patients with heart failure, diuretics and cardiotonic agent are administrated if necessary. To prevent life-threatening arrhythmia, antiarrhythmic agents are administered intravenously. If patients can visit hospital within 3 hours (ideally 1 hour) after the onset of symptoms, intravenous thrombolysis or percutaneous catheter intervention (coronary angioplasty or coronary stenting) is performed. Patient with severe multiple coronary lesions undergo coronary artery bypass grafting. In cases of severe mechanical complications such as papillary muscle rupture and ventricular septal perforation, surgical repair is performed.

vasodilator
血管拡張薬

thrombolysis
血栓溶解療法

Comprehension questions 2

1. **What are the main causes of sudden death in AMI?**

----

2. **List the medicines and surgical treatments in AMI.**

II. Vocabulary

☐ acute coronary syndrome	急性冠症候群
☐ acute myocardial infarction	急性心筋梗塞
☐ angina [pectoris]	狭心症《正式にはangina pectorisだが，臨床現場では単にanginaとされることが多い》
☐ anti-arrhythmic agent	抗不整脈薬
☐ anti-platelet agent	抗血小板薬
☐ aortic aneurysm	大動脈瘤
☐ aortic regurgitation	大動脈弁逆流〔症〕
☐ arrhythmia	不整脈
☐ aspirin	アスピリン《消炎鎮痛薬，抗血小板薬。非ステロイド系抗消炎薬の一つで成分はアセチルサリチル酸acetylsalicylic acid。Aspirinは商標名》
☐ atheroma	粥腫
☐ atrial fibrillation	心房細動
☐ atrio-ventricular block	房室ブロック
☐ bradycardia	徐脈
☐ cardiac failure, heart failure	心不全
☐ cardiac sudden death	心臓突然死
☐ cardiac tamponade	心タンポナーデ
☐ cardiogenic shock	心原性ショック
☐ cardiomyopathy	心筋症
☐ cardiotonic agent	強心薬
☐ cardiovascular disease	心血管疾患
☐ catheter intervention	カテーテル治療
☐ coronary angioplasty	冠動脈形成術
☐ coronary artery bypass graft (CABG)	冠動脈バイパス術
☐ coronary stenting	冠動脈ステント留置術
☐ deep vein thrombosis (DVT)	深部静脈血栓症
☐ diuretic	利尿薬

☐ dyslipidemia	脂質異常症	
☐ fibrous cap	線維性皮膜	
☐ infective endocarditis	感染性心内膜炎	
☐ jugular venous distension (JVD)	頸静脈怒張	
☐ mitral regurgitation	僧帽弁逆流（閉鎖不全）症	
☐ morphine	モルヒネ	
☐ myocardial infarction	心筋梗塞	
☐ myocardial ischemia	心筋虚血	
☐ nitrate	硝酸薬	
☐ papillary muscle rupture	乳頭筋断裂	
☐ percutaneous catheter intervention (PCI)	経皮的冠動脈インターベンション	
☐ risk factor	危険因子	
☐ tachycardia	頻脈	
☐ valve replacement	弁置換〔術〕	
☐ valvular heart disease	心臓弁膜症	
☐ ventricular fibrillation	心室細動	
☐ ventricular free wall rupture	〔心室〕自由壁破裂	
☐ ventricular septal perforation	心室中隔穿孔	
☐ ventricular tachycardia	心室頻拍	

III. Medical communication

Listen to the recording of the following case report and fill in the blanks. Then do the exercises that follow.

Case report

A 75-year-old man presented to our emergency department with substernal pain, _____ and occasional lightheadedness. The substernal pain had started ___ _____ earlier when eating lunch. He had been experiencing the same symptoms for the last _____. At first, he felt pain only _____, mainly when jogging. In the two weeks prior to admission, the pain had _____ and was easily induced by low level exercise, sometimes even ___ _____. He has past history of uncontrolled hypertension and _____.

On physical examination, the patient exhibited moderate distress. The patient's temperature was 37.0°C, pulse rate was _____ bpm and regular, blood pressure was _____ / _____ mmHg, and respiratory rate was 22 breaths per minute. Cardiac examination revealed a grade II/VI systolic _____ at apex and S1 and S2 were normal. There was no JVD, S3 and S4. Auscultation revealed no crackles or _____ in the lungs. The patient's ECG (Figures 1, 2) showed a sinus rhythm of 70 bpm and, ST _____ in leads II, III, aVf and V_6, and ST depression in leads V_1-V_4. Troponin T was positive with a CK of 800 IU/L and positive MB fraction.

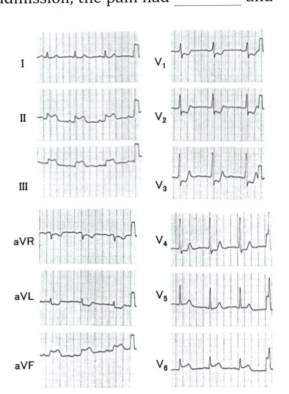

Figure 1. 12 leads ECG record on admission.

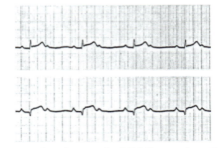

Figure 2. Record of ECG monitor in CCU (coronary care unit).

Clinical exercises

1. **What examination will be appropriate to evaluate the function of damaged organ in this case?**

   a   Abdominal CT
   b   Angiography
   c   Endoscopy
   d   Tissue biopsy
   e   Ultrasound

2. **What is the diagnosis of disease?**

   a   Gallstone
   b   Gastric ulcer
   c   Angina pectoris
   d   Acute myocardial infarction (AMI)
   e   Gastroesophageal reflux disease (GERD)

3. **What is NOT the risk factor of this disease?**

   a   Smoking
   b   Hypertension
   c   Diabetes mellitus
   d   High blood uric acid
   e   High blood HDL cholesterol

4. **What is the diagnosis of monitor ECG (Figure 2) of this patient?**

   a   Atrial flatter
   b   Atrial fibrillation
   c   Atrial premature beat
   d   Third degree atrio-ventricular block
   e   Second degree atrio-ventricular block

Check your answers.

Case report

A 75-year-old man presented to our emergency department with [1] substernal pain, **nausea** and occasional lightheadedness. The substernal pain had started **2 hours** earlier when eating lunch. He had been experiencing the same symptoms for the last **2 months**. At first, he felt pain only **occasionally,** mainly when [2] jogging. In the two weeks prior to admission, the pain had **worsened** and [3] was easily induced by low level exercise, sometimes even **at rest**. He has past history of [4] uncontrolled hypertension and **diabetes**.

On physical examination, the patient exhibited moderate distress. The patient's temperature was 37.0°C, pulse rate was **70** bpm and regular, blood pressure was **100/60** mmHg, and respiratory rate was 22 breaths per minute. [5] Cardiac examination revealed [6] a grade II/VI systolic **murmur** at apex and S1 and S2 were normal. There was no JVD, S3 and S4. Auscultation revealed no crackles or **wheezes** in the lungs. The patient's ECG showed [7] a sinus rhythm of 70 bpm and, ST **elevation** in leads II, III, aVf and V_6, and ST depression in leads V_1-V_4. Troponin T was positive with a CK of 800 IU/L and positive MB fraction.

substernal 心窩部の

lightheadedness
ふらっとする感じ

induce 誘発する

distress 苦痛

systolic 収縮期の

auscultation 聴診

CK クレアチンキナーゼ
（creatine kinase）

Note how the following common phrases are used in case reports.

・年齢，性別，主訴と随伴症状について述べる。

❶ A 75-year-old man **presented to** our emergency department with ...

（患者は75歳男性。…のため，救急外来を受診した。）

・症状の経過について述べる。

❷ At first, he felt pain only occasionally, mainly when ....

❸ In the two weeks prior to admission, the pain had worsened and ....

（最初痛みは…のとき，ごくたまに感じる程度だった。最近2週間，痛みがひどくなり，…。）

・疾患に関係しそうな既往歴について述べる。

❹ He has **past history of** ...（コントロール不良の高血圧と糖尿病の既往がある。）

・バイタルサインについて述べる。

　　バイタルサインには意識状態，体温，脈拍数と規則性，血圧，呼吸数が含まれる。また不整脈がある場合は，脈拍数と聴診で数えた心拍数の差も重要となる場合がある。

❺ The patient's **temperature** was 37.0°C, **pulse rate** was 70 bpm and regular, **blood pressure** was 100/60 mmHg, and **respiratory rate** was 22 breaths per minute.

（バイタルサインは，体温37度，脈拍数70/分（整），血圧100/60 mmHg，呼吸数22回/分。）

・診察・検査の結果について述べる。

❻ Cardiac **examination revealed** ...（心臓の診察では…を聴取し）

❼ The patient's **ECG showed** ...（心電図では…を認める。）

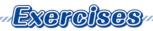

- **Write a case report of the following patient and present it in the class.**

  56歳, 男性。3カ月前からときどき起きる労作時の前胸部痛を主訴に外来を受診した。胸痛は主に階段を昇るときなどに起きるが, 最近は食後や興奮したときなどにも起きる。痛みは胸部の中央から始まり, だんだん顎や左肩から腕にも広がっていく。既往歴としては10年来の高血圧と脂質異常症がある。

IV. Further Study

Search for information about the risk factors which should be controlled to prevent acute myocardial infarction (AMI) and treatments in the acute phase of AMI. Also briefly explain the obtained information in simple English, the way you would do when talking to a patient.

A. Prevention (Risk factors)

B. Medications

C. Percutaneous coronary intervention

D. Surgical treatment

COLUMN

英文ライティングのルール ❸　スペーシング

　英単語の間をスペースで区切るのは常識ですが，英文ライティングでは日本語では使わないスペースが必要なため，日本人の落とし穴になっているケースもあります。例えば日本語では句読点やカッコは文字自体に空きスペースが含まれていますが，英語では必ずスペースを入力しなくてはいけません。

　また，数字と単位の組合せでも，日本語ではスペースを入れませんが，英語では数字と単位の間には必ずスペースが入ります。

168 cm　　55 kg　　100 mmHg

　ただし，唯一の例外が％で，この場合だけはスペースが入りません（1.0%）。また温度記号については，医学・生物学系ではスペースを入れない（37.0℃）のが慣例ですが，分野によっては入れる場合もあるようです。

　また数式を書くときも，記号の前後にはスペースを入れます（x + y = z）。

　些細なことのように思えるかもしれませんが，この点を間違えると「この著者は英語がよくわかっていない」という先入観をもたれてしまいますので，気をつけましょう。

4. Inflammatory bowel disease

　炎症性腸疾患（inflammatory bowel disease, IBD）は長期にわたり発熱・下痢・腹痛・血便などが続く原因不明の疾患です。潰瘍性大腸炎（ulcerative colitis, UC）とクローン病（Crohn's disease, CD）に大別され，どちらも現在のところ根治する治療法はなく（UCは大腸全摘という方法がありますが），厚生労働省の特定疾患にも指定されています。日本でも患者数は増加傾向にあり，今後さらなる病態解明，治療の進歩が待たれています。

Pre-reading activities

Do the following exercise before the class.

1. **What does the term "inflammatory" mean?**

2. **What are the components of the bowels?**

3. **What are the symptoms of inflammatory bowel disease?**

4. **What medications are used for inflammatory bowel disease?**

5. **How many people suffer from inflammatory bowel disease in Japan?**

I. Reading

Read the following passages and answer the questions that follow them.

Passage 1

Inflammatory bowel disease

Inflammatory bowel disease (IBD) is a broad term that describes various conditions involving chronic or recurring immune responses and inflammation of the gastrointestinal tract. The two most common inflammatory bowel diseases are ulcerative colitis and Crohn's disease. Inflammation affects the entire digestive tract in Crohn's disease but only the large intestine in ulcerative colitis. Both diseases are characterized by abnormal immune responses.

chronic 慢性の

recurring
繰り返す，再発性の

immune response
免疫反応

How does IBD occur?

In people with IBD, the immune system mistakes food, bacteria, and other materials in the intestine for invading foreign substances, and it responds by attacking the cells of the intestines. In the process, the body sends white blood cells into the lining of the intestines where they produce chronic inflammation. IBD gets worse over time and causes severe gastrointestinal symptoms that can affect patient's quality of life.

foreign substance
異物

lining 内層，内張り

Epidemiology of IBD

In the United States, 1 to 1.3 million people are estimated to suffer from IBD. The cause of the disease is unknown, and until we understand it better, it will be impossible either to prevent or cure. We do know, however, that IBD affects some subpopulations more than others. Ulcerative colitis is slightly more common in men, for example, while Crohn's disease is more frequently observed in women. As far as ethnicity is concerned, IBD occurs more in Caucasians and people of Ashkenazi Jewish origin than in other racial and ethnic subgroups. Previously noted racial

suffer from...
…を患う

subpopulation
部分母集団

Caucasian 白色人種の

Ashkenazi Jewish
アシュケナジ《ドイツ・
ポーランド・ロシア系
ユダヤ人》

46

and ethnic differences seem to be narrowing, though. Although we have only incomplete data on certain subgroups, including racial/ethnic minorities and geographic regions, reported rates remain in similar ranges.

One reason why we still do not have a precise understanding of how many people experience Crohn's disease and ulcerative colitis is that we lack standard criteria for diagnosing IBD. The criteria applied are often inconsistent, so many people with IBD may be diagnosed with other conditions.

(Adapted from: https://www.cdc.gov/ibd/what-is-ibd.htm)

racial 人種の
ethnic 民族の

Comprehension questions 1

1. How many people are estimated to suffer from IBD in USA?

2. What is the difference in the gender tendency between ulcerative colitis and Crohn's disease?

3. How are racial and ethnic differences thought to affect the prevalence of IBD?

4. Inflammatory bowel disease　47

Passage 2

Crohn's disease

Crohn's disease is a condition of chronic inflammation potentially involving any location in the gastrointestinal tract, but it most often affects the end of the small intestine and the beginning of the large intestine. In Crohn's disease, all layers of the intestine may be involved, and patches of diseased intestine can be interspersed with sections of normal healthy intestine.

Symptoms include:

- persistent diarrhea
- cramping abdominal pain
- fever
- occasional rectal bleeding

Loss of appetite and weight loss may also occur, and Crohn's disease can also affect the joints, eyes, skin, and liver. Fatigue is another common complaint.

The most common complication of Crohn's disease is blockage of the intestine due to swelling and scar tissue. Symptoms of blockage include cramping pain, vomiting, and bloating. Another complication is sores or ulcers within the intestinal tract. Sometimes these deep ulcers turn into tracts called fistulas. Patients with Crohn's disease also have an increased risk of colon cancer.

The majority of patients with Crohn's disease will require surgery at some point in their lives: surgery becomes necessary when the symptoms can no longer be controlled by medication.

Ulcerative colitis

Ulcerative colitis is a chronic gastrointestinal disorder that occurs in the top layers of the colon.

Symptoms include:

- progressive loosening of the stool*

potentially 潜在的に

intersperse 散在する

cramping 痙攣性の

progressive
進行性の

- loss of appetite and weight loss
- fatigue

*The stool is generally bloody, and patients may experience cramping abdominal pain and the need for urgent bowel movements. The onset of diarrhea may be slow or quite sudden.

Almost half of all patients with ulcerative colitis have mild symptoms. However, others may suffer from severe abdominal cramping, bloody diarrhea, nausea, and fever. The symptoms of ulcerative colitis come and go, with fairly long periods in between flare-ups.

flare-up 再発

Complications can include bleeding from deep ulcerations, rupture of the bowel, or failure to respond to the usual medical treatments. Another complication is severe abdominal bloating. Patients with ulcerative colitis are at increased risk of colon cancer.

In over a quarter of patients with ulcerative colitis, medical therapy is not completely successful and surgery may be considered to remove the colon (a procedure known as a colectomy). Ulcerative colitis is "cured" once the colon is removed.

colectomy
結腸切除術

(Adapted from: https://www.cdc.gov/ibd/what-is-ibd.htm)

Comprehension questions 2

1. List the complications of Crohn's disease.

2. List the complications of ulcerative colitis.

4. Inflammatory bowel disease　49

II. Vocabulary

☐ acute appendicitis	急性虫垂炎
☐ acute gastroenteritis	急性胃腸炎
☐ ascites	腹水
☐ cholangitis	胆管炎
☐ cholecystitis	胆嚢炎
☐ cholelithiasis	胆石症
☐ colectomy	結腸切除術
☐ colon cancer	大腸癌
☐ Crohn's disease	クローン病《口腔から肛門までの全消化管に，非連続性の慢性肉芽腫性炎症を生じる原因不明の炎症性疾患で，腹痛，下痢，体重減少，発熱，肛門病変などがよくみられる。》
☐ duodenal ulcer	十二指腸潰瘍
☐ esophageal cancer	食道癌
☐ eophageal varix, [pl.] — varices	食道静脈瘤
☐ fistula	瘻孔
☐ functional dyspepsia (FD)	機能性消化管障害
☐ gastric caner	胃癌
☐ gastric ulcer	胃潰瘍
☐ gastric varix, [pl.] — varices	胃静脈瘤
☐ gastroesophageal reflux disease (GERD)	胃食道逆流症
☐ generalized peritonitis	汎発性腹膜炎
☐ ileus	腸閉塞
☐ inflammatory bowel disease (IBD)	炎症性腸疾患《主として消化管に炎症を起こす原因不明の慢性疾患の総称で，Crohn's disease と ulcerative colitis からなり，いずれも日本では厚生労働省により特定疾患に指定されている。両疾患の違いについては本文を参照。》
☐ inguinal hernia	鼠径ヘルニア
☐ intussusception	腸重積症

☐ irritable bowel syndrome (IBS)	過敏性腸症候群
☐ laparoscope; laparoscopy	腹腔鏡；腹腔鏡検査法
☐ muscle (muscular) guarding	筋性防御
☐ pancreatic cancer	膵癌
☐ pancreatitis	膵炎
☐ peptic ulcer	消化性潰瘍
☐ peritoneal [irritation] sign	腹膜刺激徴候
☐ rupture	破裂，破綻，断裂
☐ sore	びらん
☐ ulcer	潰瘍
☐ ulceration; ulcerate	潰瘍形成；潰瘍を起こす，潰瘍化する
☐ ulcerative colitis	潰瘍性大腸炎《主に大腸粘膜に潰瘍やびらんができる原因不明の非特異性の炎症性疾患で，血便，下痢などを呈する。》

III. Medical communication

Listen to the recording of the following case report and fill in the blanks. Then do the exercises that follow.

Case report

A _____-year-old male patient presented with abdominal pain and diarrhea. The abdominal pain in the _____ _____ quadrant first appeared _____ _____ ago; he also has experienced diarrhea 5 times a day for the past week. He also noted a fever higher than _____ °C since _____.

His height is _____ cm and weight is _____ kg. He has a temperature of _____ °C, a heart rate of _____ bpm and regular, a blood pressure of _____/_____ mmHg. Physical examination revealed anemia in his palpebral conjunctiva, without jaundice. He has a palpable mass with tenderness in his right lower abdomen, without muscle guarding. The liver and the spleen are not palpable. He underwent a hemorrhoidectomy at the age of _____.

Tests revealed no anomaly in his urine. ESR _____ mm/hr, RBC _____ million/dL, Hb _____ g/dL, WBC _____ /µL, platelets _____ /µL, total protein _____ g/dL, albumin _____ g/dL. AST _____ IU/L, ALT _____ IU/L, CRP _____ mg/dL. His colonoscopy is shown in Figures 1 and 2.

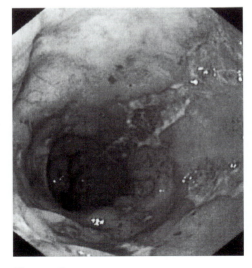

Figure 1.

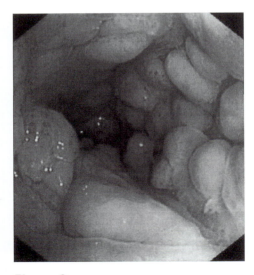

Figure 2.

Clinical exercises

1. **Which of the following is the most likely to have caused this patient's diarrhea?**

   a   hormone production

   b   decreased peristalsis

   c   enzyme deficiency

   d   bacterial toxin

   e   mucosal damage

2. **Which of the following examinations will be the most useful for diagnostic purposes? Choose two.**

   a   contrast enema of the small bowel

   b   abdominal CT

   c   abdominal radiography

   d   selective celiac angiography

   e   endoscopic ultrasonography

3. **Which of the following will be the most appropriate medication?**

   a   a laxative

   b   a chemotherapeutic agent

   c   an anticoagulant drug

   d   a corticosteroid

   e   a non-steroidal antiinflammatory drug

(Translation of part of the National Examination for Medical Practitioners 101 E19–21)

Check your answers.

Case report

A **21**-year-old male patient presented with abdominal pain and diarrhea.❶ The abdominal pain in the **right lower** quadrant first appeared **3 months** ago;❷ he also has experienced diarrhea 5 times a day for the past week. He also noted a fever higher than **37** °C since **this morning**.

His height is **168** cm and weight is **54** kg. He has a temperature of **37.2** °C, a heart rate of **72** bpm and regular, a blood pressure of **118/62** mmHg.❸ Physical examination revealed❹ anemia in his palpebral conjunctiva, without jaundice. He has a palpable mass with tenderness in his right lower abdomen, without muscle guarding. The liver and the spleen are not palpable. He underwent a hemorrhoidectomy at the age of **19**.❺

Tests revealed no anomaly in his urine. ESR **48** mm/hr, RBC **310** million/dL, Hb **9.1** g/dL, WBC **9,800**/μL, platelets **510,000**/μL, total protein **5.8** g/dL, albumin **2.3** g/dL. AST **25** IU/L, ALT **25** IU/L, CRP **3.8** mg/dL.❻ His colonoscopy is shown in Figures 1 and 2.❼

palpebral conjunctiva
眼瞼結膜

jaundice
黄染《通常は「黄疸」だが，眼科では「黄染」》

undergo
…を受ける，経験する

hemorrhoidectomy
痔核切除術

Note how the following common phrases are used in case reports.

・最初に患者の年齢・性別と主訴を述べる。

❶ A 21-year-old male patient **presented with** ...（患者は21歳，男性で…を訴えて来院した。）

・症状の経過について述べる。

❷ The abdominal pain **in the right lower quadrant** first appeared 3 months ago.（腹痛は右下腹部で，3カ月前から始まった。）

・バイタルサインについて述べる。

❸ 37.2 °C; 72 **bpm**; 118/62 **mmHg**

口頭では単位を省くことが多いが，読むときはそれぞれ下記の通り。

- 37.2 ℃ : thirty-seven **point** two **degrees Celsius**
- 72 bpm: seventy-two **beats per minute**
- 118/62 mmHg: one/a hundred (and) eighteen **over** sixty-two **millimeters of mercury**

なお英語で単位を記すときは数字と単位の間にスペースを入れる（唯一の例外は％）。

・診察所見を述べる。下記は定型表現。

❹ Physical examination **revealed** ...（身体診察で…が明らかとなった。）

・手術歴があれば述べる。

❺ He **underwent** a hemorrhoidectomy ...（痔核切除術を受けた。）

undergoは「（好ましくないことを）受ける，経験する，耐える」という意味。

・検査所見を述べる。

❻ ESR; RBC; Hb; WBC; AST; ALT; CRP

検査所見を述べる際には略語が多用される。

- **ESR:** erythrocyte sedimentation rate（赤血球沈降速度，赤沈）
- **RBC:** red blood cell (= erythrocyte)（赤血球）
- **Hb:** hemoglobin（ヘモグロビン，血色素）
- **WBC:** white blood cell (= leukocyte)（白血球）
- **AST:** aspartate aminotransferase（アスパラギン酸アミノトランスフェラーゼ；肝臓や心臓，筋肉の機能障害の指標。以前はGOT [glutamic-oxaloacetic transaminase] といわれていた）
- **ALT:** alanine aminotransferase（アラニンアミノトランスフェラーゼ；肝臓の機能障害の指標。以前はGPT [glutamic-pyruvic transaminase] といわれていた）
- **CRP:** C-reactive protein（C反応性蛋白；炎症の指標）

・検査結果を図示する。下記は定型表現。

❼ His colonoscopy **is shown in** Figures 1 and 2.

（結腸鏡による検査結果を図1，2に示す。）

4. Inflammatory bowel disease　55

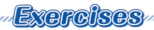

- **Write a case report on the following patient and present it in the class.**

  48歳，女性。時折起こる上腹部痛を訴えて来院。痛みは2週間前から始まった。1日に最低1回は起こり，約1時間続く。脂っこい食事で悪化し，牛乳や制酸剤を飲むと治まる。痛みの度合いは10段階評価で7。吐き気を伴うこともある。下痢や便秘はなし。体重・食欲・便の色に変化はないという。

IV. Further Study

Search for information about the treatments of inflammatory bowel disease including those under investigation (microbiome, stem cell therapy, etc) through the Internet and academic papers. Also briefly explain the obtained information in simple English, the way you would do when talking to a patient.

A. Surgery (proctocolectomy, ileostomy, colostomy, etc.)

B. Medications (mesalazine, prednisone, azathioprine, etc.)

C. Nutritional and dietetic therapies

D. Microbiome

E. Novel approaches (e.g. stem cell therapy)

4. Inflammatory bowel disease 57

COLUMN

略語のルール

　医学・医療の世界ではとても複雑で長い専門用語が多いため，略語が多用されています。例えば心肺蘇生に使うAEDの正式名称はautomated external defibrillator（自動体外式除細動器）ですが，一刻を争う緊急時に少しでも速く情報を伝えるためには略語が欠かせないことは理解できるでしょう。

　しかし一方で，違う用語が略語としては同じというケースも多々あります。例えばMSは神経科ならmultiple sclerosis（多発性硬化症），循環器科ならmitral stenosis（僧帽弁狭窄症）ですし，カルテの記載ならmorning stiffness（朝のこわばり）を意味しているかもしれません。

　近年は複数の専門領域にまたがる学際研究（multidisciplinary study）が増えていることもあって，他の分野の読者が読んでも理解できるように，略語の使用には下記のように国際的なルールが設けられています。

1．その文章の中で多用される語に限る。
2．標準的に使われている略語を用いる。
3．タイトルには略語を使わない。
4．最初にフルスペルで表記しカッコ内に略語を示す。
5．いったん略語を示したら，その後はすべて略語で示す。

　国際的な医学専門誌の編集者の団体International Committee of Medical Journal Editors（ICMJE）では，学術論文の投稿についてのガイドライン（Recommendations）を発表していますので，下記のホームページを参照してください。

ICMJE Recommendations
<http://www.icmje.org/recommendations/browse/>

5. Cirrhosis of the liver

　肝硬変 (cirrhosis of the liver) は，一つの独立した疾患というよりも，種々原因によって生じた慢性肝炎が治癒せずに長い経過をたどった後の終末像であり，その肝病変は一般的には非可逆的と考えられてきました。すなわち肝硬変とは，種々の原因によりびまん性の肝細胞の壊死と炎症・再生が繰り返し起こり，その場所に高度の線維が増生した結果，肝臓の本来の小葉構造と血管系が破壊されて偽小葉と再生結節が形成され，肝臓が萎縮し，かつ硬くなる病気です。

Pre-reading activities

Do the following exercise before the class.

1. **How can hardening and contraction of the liver be explained in histopathological terms?**

2. **What are the causes of cirrhosis?**

3. **What diseases typically cause cirrhosis in Japan? List three diseases.**

4. **What are the main symptoms of cirrhosis?**

I. Reading

Read the following passages, and answer the questions that follow them.

Passage 1

Cirrhosis is a disease in which liver cells are lost and the liver hardens. It is caused by the destruction of hepatic lobules and blood vessels and the formation of pseudolobules and regenerating nodules as the result of increased, highly dense fibrosis, where necrosis of diffuse hepatocytes and repeated inflammation-regenerations occur.

Its severity varies from almost asymptomatic at the outset to various progressive symptoms, mainly associated with deterioration of liver function due to hepatocyte damage, portal hypertension, and portosystemic shunts.

It is important to note that cirrhosis of the liver is also a systemic disease.

What causes cirrhosis?

Cirrhosis has various causes. Many patients with cirrhosis have more than one cause of liver damage.

The list below shows common causes of cirrhosis:

1) viral hepatitis (especially hepatitis C and B)
2) alcohol abuse
3) autoimmune hepatitis
4) drugs and toxic chemicals
5) cholestasis (damage, destruction, or blockage of the bile ducts)
6) liver congestion, such as right ventricular failure
7) nutritional or metabolic disorders
8) infections (including parasitic infections)

In Japan, the most common causes of cirrhosis are hepatitis C and B, followed by alcohol-related liver disease. About 80% of viral cirrhosis is caused by hepatitis C virus (HCV).

---

lobule 小葉

diffuse びまん性の

deterioration 悪化

portosystemic
門脈体静脈の

cholestasis
胆汁うっ滞

Signs and symptoms

The main symptoms of cirrhosis are caused by hepatocellular dysfunction and portal hypertension. Cirrhosis is clinically classified into a compensated period and a decompensated period, based on the presence of symptoms of liver failure without considering its cause.

Patients with compensated cirrhosis have mild or no symptoms, and no abnormality may be seen in serum chemistry tests. However, there are patients with cryptogenic cirrhosis that is found by chance.

Patients with decompensated cirrhosis have symptoms such as systemic lassitude, lack of appetite, weakness or weariness, dark urine, abdominal bloating, and nausea or vomitting. They also often complain of generalized symptoms, mainly digestive symptoms, such as abdominal pain.

However, these are not necessarily typical symptoms of cirrhosis. If the disease progresses to a severe stage, sequelae and complications such as jaundice, ascites, edema, gastrointestinal hemorrhage (hematemesis and melena), and hepatic encephalopathy (including coma) are seen. Additionally, cutaneous findings such as spider angiomas, palmar erythema, epigastric varices (Medusa's head), skin pigmentation, tendency to bleed, subcutaneous hemorrhage, clubbed fingers, and white nails as well as gynecomastia are also seen.

compensated
代償性の

cryptogenic
潜在性の，原因不明の
（＝idiopathic）

systemic
＝generalized
lassitude＝fatigue

sequela 続発症

varix 静脈瘤
Medusa's head
メデューサの頭《臍から放射状に伸びる拡張蛇行静脈》
pigmentation
色素沈着

Comprehension questions 1

1. **What are the typical clinical symptoms of cirrhosis?**

   ....

2. **What is the mechanism that causes its symptoms?**

   ....

Passage 2

How is cirrhosis diagnosed?

Cirrhosis was originally defined in histopathological terms. However, it is not easy to make a definitive diagnosis under the microscope, even after repeated laparoscopic examinations and liver biopsies, and there is no specific test. Cirrhosis is usually diagnosed comprehensively, by taking into account findings of blood chemistry, blood coagulation, and imaging tests (abdominal ultrasonography or CT) .

In its diagnosis, the following are important findings:

- increased transaminase
- elevated total bilirubin
- decreased albumin, cholinesterase, coagulation factors (prothrombin time and hepaplastin), and cholesterol
- abnormal levels of plasma-free amino acid
- increased ammonia, γ-globulin
- high scores in zinc sulfate turbidity tests (ZTT) and thymol turbidity tests (TTT)
- elevated levels of hepatic fibrosis markers
- increased levels in the indocyanine green test (15 min.)
- decreased levels of thrombocytes

In imaging tests, the following can be seen:

- irregular liver surface
- dull liver margins
- ascites
- splenomegaly

The severity of cirrhosis is a very important factor in deciding courses of treatment and advising patients about lifestyles. The Child-Pugh score is used to determine the prognosis and the necessity of liver transplantation.

Treatment for cirrhosis

Treatment depends on whether the cirrhosis is compensated

---

histopathological
組織病理学の

laparoscopic
腹腔鏡の

zinc sulfate
turbidity test
硫酸亜鉛混濁試験

thymol turbidity
test チモール混濁試験

indocyanine green
test（ICG）インドシア
ニングリーン試験

splenomegaly 脾腫

Child-Pugh score
チャイルド・ピュースコア

or decompensated. It is important to treat possible complications at an early stage and not to exacerbate current conditions, taking patients' quality of life (QOL) and activities of daily living (ADL) into account. The following elements are keys to management:

1) advice about lifestyle (including nutritional guidance)
2) commonly used medication therapy (liver support therapy)
3) antiviral therapy for viral cirrhosis (causal treatment for hepatitis C and B)
4) treatment for hepatic encephalopathy
5) liver transplantation
6) treatment for decompensated complications (jaundice, ascites, hepatic encephalopathy, gastrointestinal hemorrhage, etc.)

In Japan, there are currently many cases of living-donor liver transplantation.

Comprehension questions 2

1. **What are the most useful tests for diagnosing cirrhosis?**

2. **How does severity affect the choice of clinical treatment?**

5. Cirrhosis of the liver   63

II. Vocabulary

☐ abdominal distention	腹部膨満感
☐ alcoholic liver cirrhosis	アルコール性肝硬変
☐ autoimmune hepatitis	自己免疫性肝炎
☐ cholestatic cirrhosis	胆汁うっ滞性肝硬変《従来から使用されてきたprimary biliary cirrhosis, PBC（原発性胆汁性肝硬変）の名称が2016年4月以降，primary biliary cholangitis（原発性胆汁性胆管炎）と変更されたが，英語のprimary biliary cirrhosisの英語表記は残し，その対応する日本語は「原発性胆汁性肝硬変（旧）」と記載する》
☐ chronic hepatitis	慢性肝炎
☐ chronic liver disease	慢性肝疾患
☐ cirrhosis [of the liver]	肝硬変
☐ compensated cirrhosis	代償性肝硬変《黄疸・腹水・浮腫・肝性脳症・消化管出血など，肝機能低下と門脈圧亢進に基づく明らかな症候がいずれも認められない病態をいう》
☐ congestive cirrhosis	うっ血性肝硬変
☐ contracted liver, liver atrophy	肝臓の萎縮
☐ cryptogenic cirrhosis, idiopathic cirrhosis	潜在性肝硬変，特発性肝硬変，原因不明の肝硬変
☐ curative therapy	原因療法，根治療法
☐ decompensated cirrhosis	非代償性肝硬変
☐ epigastric varices, Medusa's head	腹壁静脈怒張，メデューサの頭
☐ esophagogastric varix, gastroesophageal varix	食道・胃静脈瘤，胃・食道静脈瘤
☐ fibrosis	線維化
☐ gastrointestinal hemorrhage, hematemesis, melena	消化管出血，吐血，下血
☐ gynecomastia	女性化乳房
☐ hardened liver	肝臓の硬化
☐ hepatic encephalopathy	肝性脳症
☐ hepatic steatosis, fatty liver	脂肪肝
☐ hypersplenism	脾機能亢進症

☐	increased fibrosis, fibrotic proliferation	線維増生
☐	jaundice	黄疸
☐	liver cancer, hepatocellular carcinoma	肝癌，肝細胞癌
☐	liver dysfunction	肝機能障害
☐	liver failure, hepatic failure	肝不全
☐	liver supporting therapy	肝庇護療法
☐	living-donor liver transplantation	生体肝移植
☐	non-alcoholic fatty liver disease (NAFLD)	非アルコール性脂肪性肝疾患
☐	non-alcoholic steatohepatitis (NASH)	非アルコール性脂肪性肝炎
☐	nutritional and metabolic disorder	栄養代謝障害
☐	nutritional therapy	栄養療法
☐	palmar erythema	手掌紅斑
☐	portal hypertension	門脈圧亢進〔症〕
☐	portosystemic shunt	門脈－大循環系短絡
☐	precancerous lesion	前癌病変《進行した慢性肝炎・肝硬変は肝細胞癌への前癌病変ともいわれている》
☐	pseudolobule	偽小葉
☐	regenerative nodule	再生結節
☐	skin pigmentation	皮膚の色素沈着
☐	spider angioma	クモ状血管腫
☐	systemic lassitude, general malaise	全身倦怠感
☐	virus-related liver cirrhosis	ウイルス性肝硬変
☐	weariness	易疲労感
☐	white nail, white claw	白色爪

5. Cirrhosis of the liver

III. Medical communication

**Listen to the recording of the following case report and fill in the blanks.
Then do the exercises that follow.**

Case report

A 61-year-old man came to the hospital accompanied by his family. His chief complaints were abdominal bloating and disturbance of _____.

Current status

He has been conscious of _____ fatigue for three months. One month ago, he noticed loss of _____ and _____ in the lower extremities. Abdominal bloating and _____ beginning 2 weeks ago made him unable to go out. This morning, he had a fever and became _____, and his family brought him to the hospital.

Past history

At age 47, he was told after his _____ physical examination that he had liver _____ and impaired glucose tolerance, but he did not seek medical help.

Lifestyle

He has smoked 20 cigarettes a day for _____ years. He is a playwright and from his youth he has often worked late at night while drinking alcohol.

Family history:

His mother died of _____ hemorrhage.

Present status

His consciousness level is I-2 by the Japan Coma Scale (JCS). His height is _____ cm, his weight 79 kg. He has a temperature of 37.9°C, a heart rate of _____ bpm and regular, a blood pressure of _____ / _____ mmHg, a respiratory rate of 16 breaths per minute, SpO_2 98% (room air). The ocular conjunctivae were _____, the palpebral conjunctivae anemic. There was a smell of ammonia on his breath. No abnormality was seen in his cardiac and respiratory sounds. The abdomen was distended, soft and _____, with no tenderness or muscle _____. Melena was found on digital rectal examination. There was no motor paralysis in the extremities, but there were edemas in the lower extremities.

Blood tests

RBC _____, Hb 8.8g/dL, Ht 27%, WBC 9,500 (band neutrophils 31%, segmented neutrophils 44%, eosinophils 1%, basophils 1%, monocytes 6%, lymphocytes ____%), platelets 90,000, PT 48%.

Blood biochemistry

Total _____ (concentration) 6.4 g/dL, albumin 2.5 g/dL, total bilirubin 6.9 mg/dL, direct bilirubin 4.7 mg/dL, AST 118 IU/L, ALT 96 IU/L, LD 377 IU/L (normal range 176 to 353), ALP 683 IU/L (normal range 115 to _____), γ-GTP 332 IU/L (normal range 8 to _____), amylase 50 IU/L (normal range 37 to 160), urea nitrogen 52 mg/dL, creatinine 1.1 mg/dL, uric acid 6.9 mg/dL, blood glucose 100 mg/dL, HbA1c 7.3% (normal range 4.6 to 6.2), total cholesterol 156 mg/dL, triglycerides 90 mg/dL, Na 131 mEq/L, K 4.5 mEq/L, Cl 96 mEq/L, CRP 2.4 mg/dL.

No abnormality in head CT. The following figure is the contrast-_____ CT of the abdomen.

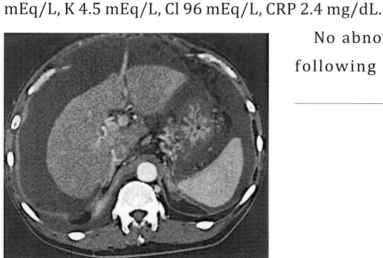

Figure 1.

Clinical exercises

1. **Which of the following conditions is the patient likely to have?**

   a nystagmus

   b orthopnea

   c nuchal rigidity

   d Babinski sign

   e asterixis (flapping tremor)

2. **Which of the following tests should be done?**

   a contrast enema

   b FDG-PET

   c cerebrospinal fluid test (CSF test)

   d lung perfusion scintigraphy

   e upper gastrointestinal endoscopy

nystagmus 眼振

orthopnea 起座呼吸

nuchal rigidity
項部硬直

flapping tremor
羽ばたき振戦

contrast enema
注腸造影

lung perfusion
scintigraphy
肺血流シンチグラフィ

(Translation of part of the National Examination for Medical Practitioners 110F 30–31)

Medical Background

肝硬変・肝癌について

・わが国では，肝癌の約60％はC型肝炎ウイルス（hepatitis C virus, HCV）感染に起因している。HCV感染は高率に持続感染を惹起し，慢性肝炎（線維化の進行を含む），肝硬変へと進行する。その後，年率7〜9％の高頻度で肝癌を発症する。一方，B型肝炎ウイルス（HBV）感染に起因する肝癌も約15％前後とほぼ一定頻度で存在する。

・わが国では，年間約3万人が肝癌により死亡している。国策が功を奏し，2005年をピークに徐々に減少しつつあり，男女合わせて死因第5番目となり，罹患数も2009年付近から減少傾向を呈しているが，5年生存率では，膵癌，胆道癌に次ぐ低い数字（約30％程度）を呈しており，さらなる対策を要する。

Check your answers.

Case report

A 61-year-old man came to the hospital accompanied by his family. ❶ His chief complaints were abdominal bloating ❷ and disturbance of **consciousness**.

chief complaint
主訴

Current status

He has been conscious of **generalized** fatigue for three months. One month ago, he noticed loss of **appetite** and **edema** in the lower extremities. Abdominal bloating and **lightheadedness** beginning 2 weeks ago made him unable to go out. This morning, he had a fever and became **drowsy**, and his family brought him to the hospital.

be aware of ...
...を自覚していた

lightheadedness
ふらつき

drowsy 傾眠状態の

Past history

At age 47, he was told after his **comprehensive** physical examination that he had liver **dysfunction** and impaired glucose tolerance, but he did not seek medical help. ❸

comprehensive physical examination 総合的健康診断，人間ドック

liver dysfunction
肝機能障害

impaired glucose tolerance
耐糖能異常

Lifestyle

He has smoked 20 cigarettes a day for **40** years. He is a playwright and from his youth he has often worked late at night while drinking alcohol.

playwright 脚本家

Family history

His mother died of **cerebral** hemorrhage.

cerebral hemorrhage 脳出血

Present status

His consciousness level is I-2 by the Japan Coma Scale (JCS). His height is **169** cm, his weight 79 kg. He has a

consciousness level 意識レベル

JCS = Japan Coma Scale

5. Cirrhosis of the liver   69

temperature of 37.9 °C, a heart rate of **84** bpm and regular, a blood pressure of **134/78** mmHg, a respiratory rate of 16 breaths per minute, SpO$_2$ 98% (room air). The ocular conjunctivae were **icteric**, the palpebral conjunctivae anemic.❹ There was a smell of ammonia on his breath. No abnormality was seen in his cardiac and respiratory sounds. The abdomen was distended, soft and **fluctuated**, with no tenderness or muscle **guarding**.❺ Melena was found on digital rectal examination. There was no motor paralysis in the extremities, but there were edemas in the lower extremities.

Blood tests

RBC **3,280,000**, Hb 8.8g/dL, Ht 27%, WBC 9,500 (band neutrophils 31%, segmented neutrophils 44%, eosinophils 1%, basophils 1%, monocytes 6%, lymphocytes **17**%), platelets 90, 000, PT 48%.

Blood biochemistry

Total **protein** (concentration) 6.4 g/dL, albumin 2.5 g/dL, total bilirubin 6.9 mg/dL, direct bilirubin 4.7 mg/dL, AST 118 IU/L, ALT 96 IU/L, LD❻ 377 IU/L (normal range 176 to 353), ALP 683 IU/L (normal range 115 to **359**), γ-GTP 332 IU/L (normal range 8 to **50**), amylase 50 IU/L (normal range 37 to 160), urea nitrogen 52 mg/dL, creatinine 1.1 mg/dL, uric acid 6.9 mg/dL, blood glucose 100 mg/dL, HbA1c 7.3% (normal range 4.6 to 6.2), total cholesterol 156 mg/dL, triglycerides 90 mg/dL, Na 131 mEq/L, K 4.5 mEq/L, Cl 96 mEq/L, CRP 2.4 mg/dL.

No abnormality in head CT. The following figure is the contrast-**enhanced** CT of the abdomen.

---

conjunctiva
眼球結膜

palpebral conjunctiva
眼瞼結膜

ammonia smell
アンモニア臭

fluctuated
波動を認める

tenderness 圧痛

digital rectal examination
直腸指診

melena 黒色便

motor paralysis
運動麻痺

edema in the lower extremities
下腿浮腫

band neutrophil
桿状核好中球

segmented neutrophil
分葉核好中球

eosinophil 好酸球

basophil 好塩基球

Note how the following common phrases are used in case reports.

❶ ... accompanied by his/her family（家族に連れられて）

be taken by the family でもよいが，accompany のほうがフォーマルな表現。

❷ distention; bloating; swelling

「膨張，腫れ」に相当する代表的な語は上の3つで，左から順に，よりフォーマルな表現。動詞は distend, bloat, swell 。逆の「縮む」は contract, shrink などが，「へこむ」は dent, cave などがある。

❸ ..., but he did not seek medical help.（医療機関を未受診であった。）

❹ The ocular conjunctivae were icteric, the palpebral conjunctivae were anemic.（眼球結膜に黄染を認め，眼瞼結膜は貧血様。）

❺ The abdomen was distended, soft and fluctuated, with no tenderness or muscle guarding.（腹部は膨隆しているが軟で，波動を認めるが，圧痛と筋性防御を認めない。）

❻ LD, ALP, γ-GTP, HbA1c

検査所見を述べる際には略語が多用される。本シナリオ関連の略語は下記の通り。

- **LD/LDH**: lactate dehydrogenase（乳酸脱水素酵素）
- **ALP**: alkaline phosphatase（アルカリホスファターゼ；肝・胆道疾患，骨疾患で数値が上昇する）
- **γ-GTP**: γ-glutamyl transferase/transpeptidase（γ-グルタミルトランスフェラーゼ／トランスペプチダーゼ；肝細胞障害，胆管障害，アルコール肝障害などの際に上昇し，肝疾患の指標となる）
- **HbA1c**: hemoglobin A1c（過去の平均血糖の指標として用いられる）

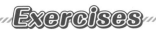

- **Write case reports on the following patients and present them in the class.**

  A．55歳，男性。全身倦怠感と軽度の食思不振を訴えて来院した。症状は約1年半前から継続している。このため仕事への集中力も低下してきている。約半年前から嗜好の変化も出現してきており，両側手掌の特に親指側と小指側が紅い。さらに，両側の手指が太鼓のばち状を呈し，両側乳房も女性様腫大を認める。皮膚にも色素沈着を認める。体重は約1.5kg減少したものの，両側下腿に浮腫を認めない。また，神経学的異常所見も認めない。なお，本患者は約20年前から近医でHCV持続感染を指摘されている。

  B．74歳，女性。身長165 cm，体重58 kg。脈拍70回/分 整，体温36.5℃，血圧137/77 mmHg，意識清明。身体診察では心窩部にやや硬度な肝を3横指触知し，左季肋部に脾を2横指触知する。腹部は平坦で波動は認めない。末梢血液検査値は，白血球3,300/μL，赤血球350万/μL，血小板7万/μL。血液生化学的検査値の主なものは，総ビリルビン1.5mg/dL，血清アルブミン3.0 g/dL，血清総コレステロール130 mg/dL，AST 50 IU/L，ALT 45 IU/L，プロトロンビン時間（PT）70％。血中アンモニア40 μg/dL。HCV-RNA：6.7 logIU/mL。

IV. Further Study

Search for information about chronic liver diseases (including chronic hepatitis and cirrhosis) through the Internet and academic papers. Also briefly explain the obtained information in simple English, the way you would do when talking to a patient.

A. Recently developed treatments for chronic hepatitis C

B. Recently developed treatments for chronic hepatitis B

C. Information about non-alcoholic fatty liver disease (NAFLD) and non-alcoholic steatohepatitis (NASH)

D. Mechanism of hepatocarcinoma in hepatitis C

E. Predispositions to hepatocarcinoma (such as hepatitis C and B)

COLUMN

イギリス英語とアメリカ英語

　同じ英語でも，イギリスとアメリカではさまざまな違いがあります。現在の日本ではアメリカ英語が主流ですが，英連邦の国々やヨーロッパではイギリス英語が主流です。文法や発音にも違いがありますが，ここでは医学に関わる単語の違いを中心にご紹介しましょう。海外の文献を読むとき，特にイギリスの学術誌では上記のようなスペルを見ることも多いと思いますが，間違いではありませんので頭に入れておきましょう。

- ●語尾：–er（米）と –re（英）
  - meter　　metre
- ●語尾：–ze（米）と –se（英）
  - analyze　　analyse
- ●語尾：–or（米）と –our（英）
  - tumor　　tumour
- ●母音：a（米）と　ae（英）
  - anemia　　anaemia
- ●母音：o（米）と　oe（英）
  - diarrhea　　diarrhoea
  - estrogen　　oestrogen

6. Rheumatoid arthritis and systemic lupus erythematosus

　関節リウマチ (rheumatoid arthritis, RA) は全身の関節に痛みと腫脹を生じ，次第に関節の破壊や変形をきたす病気です。全身性エリテマトーデス (systemic lupus erythematosus, SLE, lupus) は自己免疫現象により全身の多臓器を侵す病気です。RAおよびSLEは全身に影響が及ぶ全身性自己免疫疾患である膠原病の代表的疾患です。

Pre-reading activities

Do the following exercise before the class.

1. Define "autoimmune disease" and list a few examples besides rheumatoid arthritis (RA) and systemic lupus erythematosus (SLE).

2. Which gender and age groups is RA likely to affect?

3. What medications are often used to treat RA?

4. What are the major symptoms of SLE?

5. What organs are often affected by SLE?

I. Reading

Read the following passages, and answer the questions that follow them.

Passage 1

What is rheumatoid arthritis?

Rheumatoid arthritis is an inflammatory disease that causes[1] pain, swelling, stiffness, and loss of function in the joints. It can cause mild to severe symptoms. Rheumatoid arthritis not only affects[2] the joints, but may also attack[3] tissue in the skin, lungs, eyes, and blood vessels. Rheumatoid arthritis is classified as an autoimmune disease. An autoimmune disease occurs[4] when the immune system turns against parts of the body it is designed to protect.

loss of function
機能喪失

mild 軽度の

severe
深刻な，重症の

What happens in rheumatoid arthritis?

Rheumatoid arthritis is primarily a disease of the joints. The joint capsule is lined with a type of tissue called synovium, which produces synovial fluid, a clear substance that lubricates and nourishes the cartilage and bones inside the joint capsule.

be lined with ...
...で裏打ちされている

lubricate
滑らかにする

Like many other rheumatic diseases, rheumatoid arthritis is an autoimmune disease, so called because a person's immune system, which normally helps protect the body from infection and disease, attacks joint tissues for unknown reasons. White blood cells, the agents of the immune system, travel to the synovium and cause inflammation (synovitis), characterized by warmth, redness, swelling, and pain—typical symptoms of rheumatoid arthritis. During the inflammation process, the normally thin synovium becomes thick and makes the joint swollen, puffy, and sometimes warm to the touch.

immune system
免疫機構

puffy むくんだ

As rheumatoid arthritis progresses,[5] the inflamed synovium invades[6] and destroys the cartilage and bone within the joint. The surrounding muscles, ligaments, and tendons that support and stabilize the joint become weak and unable to work normally. These effects lead to the pain and joint damage often seen in rheumatoid arthritis. Researchers studying rheumatoid arthritis now believe that it begins to damage bones during the first year or two that a person has the disease, which is one reason why early diagnosis and treatment are so important.

> early diagnosis and treatment
> 早期診断と治療

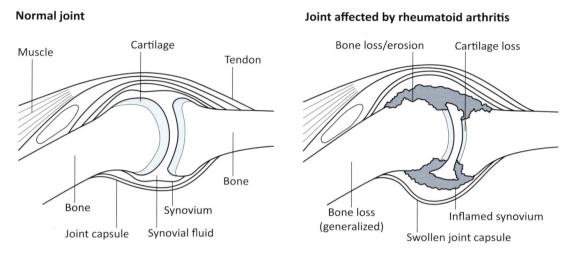

Figure 1.　The joint affected by rheumatoid arthritis.

Comprehension questions 1

1. What is the cause of autoimmune diseases?

2. What effects does rheumatoid arthritis have on the joints?

3. Why are early diagnosis and treatment of rheumatoid arthritis so important?

Passage 2

What is lupus?

Lupus is one of autoimmune diseases, in which the immune system turns against parts of the body it is designed to protect.[7] This leads to inflammation and damages[8] various body tissues. Lupus can affect many parts of the body, including the joints, skin, kidneys, heart, lungs, blood vessels, and brain.

Typically, lupus is characterized by periods of illness, called flares, and periods of wellness, or remission. Understanding how to prevent flares and how to treat them when they do occur helps people with lupus maintain better health.

Symptoms of lupus

Each person with lupus has slightly different symptoms that can range from mild to severe and may come and go over time. However, some of the most common symptoms of lupus include painful or swollen joints (arthritis), unexplained fever, and extreme fatigue. A characteristic red skin rash—the so-called butterfly or malar rash—may appear[9] across the nose and cheeks. Rashes may also occur on the face and ears, upper arms, shoulders, chest, and hands and other areas exposed to the sun. Because many people with lupus are sensitive to sunlight (a condition called photosensitivity), skin rashes often first develop or worsen[10] after sun exposure.

Other symptoms of lupus include chest pain, hair loss, anemia, mouth ulcers, and pale or purple fingers and toes caused by cold and stress. Some people also experience headaches, dizziness, depression, confusion, or seizures. New symptoms may continue to appear years after the initial diagnosis, and different symptoms can occur at different times. In some people with lupus, only one system of the body, such as the skin or joints, is affected. Other people experience symptoms in many parts of their body. Just how seriously a body system is affected varies from person to person.

(https://www.niams.nih.gov/Health_Info/Lupus/default.asp)

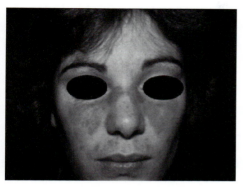

Figure 2. Malar (butterfly) rash.

(https://www.ncbi.nlm.nih.gov/pmc/articles/PMC3410306/figure/fig1/)

Comprehension questions 2

1. **List the symptoms of lupus.**

2. **What effect does exposure to sunlight have on people with lupus ?**

II. Vocabulary

☐ ankylosing spondylitis	強直性脊椎炎
☐ anti-nuclear antibody (ANA)	抗核抗体
☐ arthritis	関節炎
☐ Behçet's disease	ベーチェット病
☐ butterfly rash	蝶形紅斑
☐ disease-modifying anti-rheumatic drug (DMARD)	抗リウマチ薬
☐ eosinophilic granulomatosis with polyangiitis (EGPA), Churg-Strauss syndrome	好酸球性多発血管炎性肉芽腫症, チャーグ・ストラウス症候群
☐ fibromyalgia	線維筋痛症
☐ granulomatosis with polyangiitis (GPA), Wegener's granulomatosis	多発血管炎性肉芽腫症, ウェゲナー肉芽腫
☐ Henoch-Schönlein purpura	ヘノッホ・シェーンライン紫斑病
☐ immunosuppressant	免疫抑制薬
☐ joint erosion	関節のびらん
☐ joint space narrowing	関節裂隙の狭小化
☐ joint swelling	関節腫脹
☐ joint tenderness	関節圧痛
☐ microscopic polyangiitis (MPA)	顕微鏡的多発血管炎
☐ mixed connective disease (MCTD)	混合性結合組織病
☐ morning stiffness	朝のこわばり
☐ non-steroidal anti-inflammatory drug (NSAID)	非ステロイド性抗炎症薬
☐ osteoarthritis (OA)	変形性関節症
☐ osteoporosis	骨粗鬆症
☐ overlap syndrome	オーバーラップ症候群

☐	photosensitivity	光線過敏，日光過敏
☐	polyarteritis nodosa	結節性多発動脈炎
☐	polymyalgia rheumatica (PMR)	リウマチ性多発筋痛症
☐	polymyositis/dermatomyositis (PM/ DM)	多発性筋炎/皮膚筋炎
☐	pseudogout	偽痛風
☐	psoriatic arthritis	乾癬性関節炎
☐	Raynaud phenomenon	レイノー現象
☐	rheumatoid arthritis (RA)	関節リウマチ
☐	rheumatoid nodule	リウマチ結節
☐	sarcoidosis	サルコイドーシス
☐	scleroderma/systemic sclerosis (SSc)	強皮症/全身性硬化症
☐	Sjögren syndrome	シェーグレン症候群
☐	systemic lupus erythematosus (SLE)	全身性エリテマトーデス，ループス
☐	Takayasu arteritis	高安動脈炎
☐	temporal arteritis, giant cell arteritis	側頭動脈炎，巨細胞性動脈炎

III. Medical communication

Listen to the recording of the following case report and fill in the blanks. Then do the exercises that follow.

Case report

A _____-year-old female with depression presented to the rheumatology clinic with complaints of chronic _____ _____. She describesd suffering for _____ from multiple site _____, but had not previously sought medical attention. She also reported _____ _____ in both hands and occasionally used over-the-counter _____ _____ as needed. She denied _____ of _____. A review of systems was positive for generalized _____.

On examination, lungs were clear to auscultation bilaterally, and heart sounds were regular rate and rhythm without murmurs. Extremity exam revealed rheumatoid arthritis _____ of finger joints.

Laboratory analysis revealed mild inflammation with an elevated CRP (C-reactive protein) level of _____ mg/dL and ESR of _____ mm/hr. ANA (antinuclear antibody) was _____ and RF (rheumatoid factor) was _____. Plain-film radiographs of both hands showed changes consistent with advanced-stage rheumatoid arthritis.

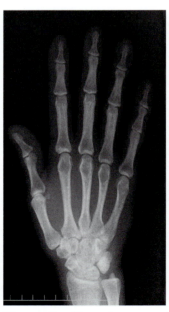 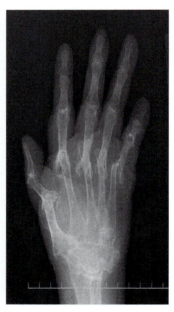

Figure 3. X-ray images of the hand.
Normal (left) and advanced stage of rheumatoid arthritis (right).

She was diagnosed with _____ _____. Treatment includes _____ _____, NSAIDs (nonsteroidal anti-inflammatory drugs), and DMARDs (disease-modifying anti-rheumatic drugs). She was also referred to a psychotherapist for her mood disorder.

Clinical exercises

1. **Which of the following laboratory tests is NOT appropriate for patients suspected of having rheumatoid arthritis?**

   a Rheumatoid factor (RF)
   b Anti-CCP antibody
   c MMP3
   d CRP
   e Anti-DNA antibody

2. **Which of the following examinations are useful for diagnosing rheumatoid arthritis? Choose two.**

   a Ultrasound
   b MRI
   c Endoscopy
   d Lumbar puncture
   e Angiography

3. **Which parts of the body are most often affected by rheumatoid arthritis?**

   a Shoulder joints
   b Wrist and finger joints
   c Ankle and toe joints
   d Hip joints
   e Spine

Check your answers.

Case report

A **68**-year-old female with depression presented to the rheumatology clinic with complaints of chronic **joint pain**. She described suffering for **decades** from multiple site **arthralgia**, but had not previously sought medical attention. She also reportd **morning stiffness** in both hands and occasionally used over-the-counter **pain medication** as needed. She denied **loss** of **weight**. A review of systems was positive for generalized **fatigue**.

On examination, lungs were clear to auscultation bilaterally, and heart sounds were regular rate and rhythm without murmurs. Extremity exam revealed rheumatoid arthritis **deformities** of finger joints.

Laboratory analysis revealed mild inflammation with an elevated CRP (C-reactive protein) level of **1.5** mg/dL and ESR of **46** mm/hr. ANA (antinuclear antibody) was **negative** and RF (rheumatoid factor) was **positive**. Plain-film radiographs of both hands showed changes consistent with advanced-stage rheumatoid arthritis.

She was diagnosed with **rheumatoid arthritis**. Treatment includes **physical therapy**, NSAIDs (nonsteroidal anti-inflammatory drugs), and DMARDs (disease-modifying anti-rheumatic drugs). She was also referred to a psychotherapist for her mood disorder.

---

a review of systems
系統的レビュー《全身スクリーニング目的のチェックリスト》

plain-film radiograph
単純X線写真

advanced-stage
進行期の

anti-inflammatory drug 抗炎症薬

psychotherapist
サイコセラピスト《精神科医，心理学者，臨床心理士，カウンセラーなどが含まれる》

Note the verbs appeared in the Reading section, which are commonly used to describe diseases.

❶ cause:〔病気・症状を〕引き起こす

Rheumatoid arthritis **causes** pain in the joints.

（関節リウマチは関節に痛みを引き起こす。）

❷ affect:〔体の部位を〕侵す，罹患する

Rheumatoid arthritis **affects** the joints.（関節リウマチは関節を侵す。）

❸ attack:〔体の部位を〕攻撃する，冒す，襲う

Rheumatoid arthritis may **attack** tissue in the skin.

（関節リウマチは皮膚の組織を冒すことがある。）

❹ occur:〔病気・症状が〕起こる

An autoimmune disease **occurs**.（自己免疫疾患が起こる。）

❺ progress:〔病気が〕進行する

Rheumatoid arthritis **progresses**.（関節リウマチが進行する。）

❻ invade:〔体の部位を〕侵す

The inflamed synovium **invades** the cartilage of the joint.

（炎症した滑膜が関節の軟骨を侵す。）

❼ protect A from B: AをBから守る

Person's immune system helps **protect** the body **from** infection.

（ヒトの免疫機構は感染から身体を守るのを助ける。）

❽ damage:〔体の部位を〕破壊する

The inflamed synovium **damages** the cartilage of the joint.

（炎症した滑膜が関節の軟骨を破壊する。）

❾ appear:〔症状が〕出現する

The so-called butterfly may **appear**.（いわゆる蝶形紅斑が出現することがある。）

❿ worsen:〔症状が〕増悪する

Skin rashes **worsen**.（皮疹が増悪する。）

6. Rheumatoid arthritis and systemic lupus erythematosus

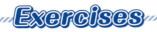

- **Write a case report on the following patient and present it in the class.**

  40歳，女性。これまで特に既往歴はない。4カ月前からの発熱のため来院。口内炎，頬の発疹，多発性関節痛が2カ月間あり。1カ月前の健診で汎血球減少と尿蛋白を指摘された。昨日かかりつけ医を受診し，風邪と診断された。日光過敏症あり，全身倦怠感あり，胸痛あり，咳嗽なし，呼吸困難なし。

IV. Further Study

Search for information about the diagnosis and medication of rheumatoid arthritis and systemic lupus erythematosus through the Internet and academic papers. Also briefly explain the obtained information in simple English, the way you would do when talking to a patient.

A. How to diagnose RA (symptoms, laboratory tests, imaging studies, etc.)

B. Medications for RA (corticosteroid, methotrexate, biologics such as TNF inhibitors, etc.)

C. How to diagnose SLE (symptoms, laboratory tests, etc.)

D. Briefly explain various symptoms and signs seen SLE patients.

6. Rheumatoid arthritis and systemic lupus erythematosus 87

COLUMN

覚えておきたい複数形

　医学用語にはラテン語やギリシャ語に由来する名詞が多数あり，そうした用語が複数形になるときは，単純に—sとはならずに，元の言語の規則を残している場合が多々あります．代表的な規則と例を紹介します．

ギリシャ語起源の単数形/複数形

–is / –es	analysis / analyses
	crisis / crises
	diagnosis / diagnoses
–itis / –itides	gastritis / gastritides
–ma / –mata	carcinoma / carcinomata
–on / –a	criterion / criteria
–osis / –oses	adenosis / adenoses

ラテン語起源の単数形/複数形

–a / –ae	ameba / amebae
	vertebra / vertebrae
-ex / –ices	apex / apices
	index / indices
–um / –a	bacterium / bacteria
	datum / data
–us / –i	bacillus / bacilli
	locus / loci
	focus / foci
	stimulus / stimuli

　「バクテリア」や「データ」など日本語になっていることばもありますが，英語でbacteriasやdatasはありえません．もともと複数形だということを覚えておきましょう．

7. Diabetes mellitus

　糖尿病 (diabetes mellitus) は，インスリンの分泌障害や抵抗性亢進などによりインスリンの作用が不足し，細胞へのブドウ糖 (＝血糖, glucose) の取り込みが減るために，血糖値が正常よりも高い状態が続く疾患です。高血糖そのものも，多尿，多飲，口渇などの症状を引き起こしますが，アシドーシスや合併症のコントロールがより重要となる疾患です。

Pre-reading activities

Do the following exercise before class.

1. **Define diabetes mellitus.**

2. **What are the major types of diabetes mellitus?**

3. **What hormones regulate blood glucose levels?**

4. **What are the symptoms, signs and complications of diabetes mellitus?**

5. **What drugs are used for diabetes mellitus?**

I. Reading

Read the following passages, and answer the questions that follow them.

Passage 1

Diabetes mellitus, commonly referred to as diabetes, is a disease characterized by high blood glucose levels (hyperglycemia). Insulin is the only hormone that reduces the blood glucose level, while a number of hormones (e.g. glucagon, catecholamine) increase it. Glucose is the main source of energy for cells. Insulin, which is made by β cells in the pancreatic islet, helps blood glucose get into cells to be used for energy. Insulin also suppresses gluconeogenesis in the liver, thereby lowering the blood glucose level. In a patient with diabetes mellitus, the pancreas does not make enough insulin and/or the cells cannot use it. As a result, hyperglycemia occurs. Over time, hyperglycemia can cause various health problems.

hyperglycemia
高血糖

suppress
抑制する

Types of diabetes mellitus

The common types of diabetes mellitus are type 1 and type 2.

Type 1 diabetes mellitus

Type 1 diabetes mellitus (DM) is characterized by deficient insulin production and requires daily administration of insulin. Therefore, type 1 DM is called insulin-dependent DM (IDDM). Although the cause of type 1 DM is not fully understood, it is thought that the immune system may attack and destroy the β cells in the pancreatic islet.

deficient 不足した

daily
administration
日々の摂取

Type 2 diabetes mellitus

Type 2 DM is the most common type of diabetes (about 95 percent of cases of adult DM). This type of diabetes basically results from the body's ineffective use of insulin. Hence, it is formally called non-insulin-dependent DM (NIDDM). Hyperglycemia in type 2 DM results from both impaired

90

insulin secretory response to glucose and decreased insulin effectiveness in stimulating glucose uptake by cells, and in inhibiting hepatic gluconeogenesis. Type 2 DM is largely the result of excess body weight and physical inactivity.

inhibit 抑制する

Comprehension questions 1

1. **Which of the following is NOT true?**

   a Diabetes mellitus is defined as too much insulin in your blood stream.

   b Type 1 diabetes is thought to be caused by the autoimmune destruction of β cells.

   c You are at increased risk of developing type 2 diabetes if you are inactive and overweight.

2. **Which of the following is NOT true?**

   a Type 1 diabetes is the most common form of diabetes.

   b In type 1 diabetes, the body does not produce enough insulin.

   c Insulin causes blood glucose levels to fall, but glucagon causes them to rise.

Passage 2

Symptoms and signs of DM

Polyuria, polydipsia and weight loss occur when hyperglycemia causes glucosuria and osmotic diuresis. Hyperglycemia also causes blurred vision, fatigue, and nausea. In type 1 DM, these symptoms may occur suddenly. The signs and symptoms of type 2 DM may be similar to those of type 1 DM, but are often less marked. Type 2 DM is frequently found in asymptomatic patients through routine health examinations and may be diagnosed several years after onset, once complications have already arisen.

blurred vision
かすみ目

asymptomatic
無症状の

7. Diabetes mellitus   91

Diabetic ketoacidosis (DKA)

Diabetic ketoacidosis (DKA) is a metabolic acidosis due to the accumulation of ketones caused by severe insulin deficiency, and it is usually observed in type 1 DM. DKA is characterized by nausea, vomiting, abdominal pain, the smell of acetone on the breath, deep breathing known as Kussmaul breathing and, in severe cases, a decreased level of consciousness.

Complications of DM

Late complications occur after several years of hyperglycemia. Microvascular complications include retinopathy, nephropathy and peripheral and autonomic neuropathy. Macrovascular complications include atherosclerotic coronary and peripheral arterial disease.

Adults with diabetes have a 2- to 3-fold increased risk of heart attacks and strokes.

Retinopathy

Diabetic retinopathy occurs as a result of long-term accumulated damage to the small blood vessels in the retina. The initial retinal change seen in DM does not significantly alter vision, but it can progress to retinal detachment or hemorrhage, which can cause blindness.

Nephropathy

Diabetes is among the leading causes of renal failure. Microalbuminuria leads to diabetic nephropathy, which is asymptomatic in the early stages. Without adequate treatment, it progresses slowly and finally causes renal insufficiency requiring renal dialysis. Diabetic nephropathy increases the risk of end-stage renal disease (ESRD) and mortality.

Neuropathy

Diabetic neuropathy commonly occurs as a distal, symmetric, predominantly sensory polyneuropathy. The sensory deficits are usually marked by a stocking-glove distribution. The neuropathy may cause numbness, tingling and paresthesia in the extremities. Autonomic disturbance (e.g. orthostatic hypotension, neurogenic bladder, and erectile dysfunction) also occurs in diabetic neuropathy. Combined with reduced blood flow, neuropathy in the feet increases the chance of foot ulcers, infection and the eventual need for limb amputation.

distal 遠位の
symmetric 対称的な
polyneuropathy
多発性神経障害
paresthesia
感覚異常
orthostatic
hypotension
起立性低血圧
neurogenic
bladder
神経因性膀胱障害
erectile
dysfunction
勃起障害
amputation 切断

Comprehension questions 2

1. **What are the three main microvascular complications of diabetes?**

2. **List three types of autonomic problems encountered in diabetic neuropathy.**

3. **List two causes of visual loss due to diabetic retinopathy.**

II. Vocabulary

☐ C peptide immunoreactivity (CPR)	Cペプチド免疫活性
☐ casual plasma (blood) glucose	随時血糖
☐ continuous subcutaneous insulin infusion	持続皮下インスリン注入療法
☐ diabetes insipidus	尿崩症
☐ diabetes mellitus, diabetes	糖尿病
☐ diabetic coma	糖尿病〔性〕昏睡
☐ diabetic foot	糖尿病足病変
☐ diabetic glomerulosclerosis	糖尿病性糸球体硬化症
☐ diabetic ketoacidosis	糖尿病〔性〕ケトアシドーシス
☐ diet therapy	食事療法
☐ dipeptidyl peptidase IV (DPP-4) inhibitor	ジペプチジル・ペプチダーゼIV阻害薬
☐ exercise therapy	運動療法
☐ fasting hyperglycemia	空腹時高血糖
☐ fasting plasma (blood) glucose (FPG, FBG)	空腹時血糖
☐ gangrene	壊疽
☐ gestational diabetes	妊娠糖尿病
☐ glucagon test	グルカゴン負荷試験
☐ glucagon-like peptide 1 (GLP-1)	グルカゴン様ペプチド
☐ glucose transporter (GLUT)	糖輸送担体
☐ glucotoxicity	糖毒性《インスリン分泌能の低下や末梢組織でのインスリン抵抗性の増大によって生じた高血糖が，さらにこれらのインスリン作用不全を増悪させ，さらなる高血糖を引き起こすことで，糖尿病の進行に深く関与している》
☐ glycolysis system	解糖系
☐ glyconeogenesis	糖新生《血糖値が低下したとき，肝臓で糖以外の材料から新たにブドウ糖を合成し，不足分を補うこと。筋からのアミノ酸，ピルビン酸，乳酸や，脂肪組織からのグリセロールなどが用いられる》

☐ hemoglobin A1c (HbA1c)	糖化ヘモグロビン	
☐ hyperosmolar hyperglycemic syndrome (HHS)	高浸透圧高血糖症候群《2型糖尿病の高齢者でしばしばみられる病態で，血糖および血液浸透圧の著明な上昇，高度な脱水を特徴とし，これらによって意識障害やけいれんなどが生じる。糖尿病性ケトアシドーシスとは異なり，ケトアシドーシスはあっても軽度》	
☐ immunoreactive insulin	免疫反応性インスリン	
☐ impaired fasting glycemia (IFG)	空腹時血糖異常	
☐ impaired glucose tolerance (IGT)	耐糖能異常	
☐ incretin	インクレチン	
☐ insulin analog	インスリンアナログ	
☐ insulin resistance	インスリン抵抗性《組織でのインスリンの感受性が低下して効きにくくなることによって，ブドウ糖の細胞への取り込みが減るために高血糖をきたす状態。インスリン抵抗性が生じる原因には，過食や運動不足など生活習慣が大きく関わっている》	
☐ insulin therapy	インスリン療法	
☐ insulin-dependent diabetes mellitus (IDDM)	インスリン依存性糖尿病	
☐ Kussmaul breathing	クスマウル呼吸《糖尿病性ケトアシドーシスによる昏睡などにみられる異常に深く規則的な呼吸》	
☐ neovascularization	血管新生	
☐ neurogenic bladder	神経因性膀胱	
☐ oral glucose tolerance test (OGTT)	経口ブドウ糖負荷試験《75 gのブドウ糖を経口投与して，食後高血糖を捉えるための検査。空腹時高血糖を示さない軽度の糖代謝異常を発見するために重要》	
☐ oral hypoglycemic agent	経口血糖降下薬	
☐ osmotic diuresis	浸透圧利尿	
☐ pancreatic islet transplantation	膵島移植	
☐ perception disorder	感覚障害	
☐ polydipsia	多飲	

7. Diabetes mellitus　95

☐ polyuria	多尿	
☐ postprandial hyperglycemia	食後高血糖	
☐ proliferative diabetic retinopathy (PDR)	増殖糖尿病網膜症	
☐ renal glycosuria (glucosuria)	腎性糖尿	
☐ retinal photocoagulation therapy	網膜光凝固療法	
☐ self-monitoring of blood glucose (SMBG)	血糖自己測定	
☐ sodium glucose cotransporter (SGLT)	ナトリウム・グルコース共輸送担体	
☐ sulfonylurea	スルホニル尿素	
☐ traction retinal detachment	牽引性網膜剥離	
☐ uremia	尿毒症	
☐ urinary glucose	尿糖	
☐ urinary microalubmin	尿中微量アルブミン	
☐ α-glucosidase inhibitor	α グルコシダーゼ阻害薬	

Table 1. Classification of oral anti-diabetic drugs.

Insulin secretagogues	Sulfonylureas	Stimulate insulin secretion from beta cells
	Meglitinides	
	Dipeptidyl peptidase-4 (DPP-4) inhibitors	
Insulin sensitizers	Biguanides	Enhance insulin sensitivity
	Thiazolidinedione (TZDs)	
Enzyme inhibitors	Alpha glucosidase inhibitors	Inhibit the breakdown of carbohydrates in the gut
	Sodium-glucose transport protein (SGLT2) inhibitors	Inhibit the reabsorption of glucose in the kidney

III. Medical communication

Listen to the conversation between a doctor and a patient and fill in the blanks. Then do the exercises that follow.

Doctor-patient conversation

A 59-year-old male patient visits a specialist for advice concerning the results of a recent health check-up.

D: Good morning. What's brought you here today?

P: Well, doctor, I had a regular check-up last week, and there seems to be a problem with my _____ _____.

D: Have you ever been diagnosed with _____?

P: No, never. But my doctor once said my blood was denser than normal. He said it was probably because I _____.

D: I see. (*He looks at the results.*) Actually, according to these results, it's your HbA1c level that's high, not the hemoglobin level. And your _____ blood glucose is _____ mg/dL. That's above normal.

P: What's the difference between HbA1c and hemoglobin?

D: Well, the HbA1c level indicates the glucose level in the blood, so it's used to diagnose _____ _____.

P: Diabetes? I've never been diagnosed with diabetes.

D: (*He checks the past data.*) Well, your HbA1c level was around five in past years. Have there been any changes in your _____ since last year? Especially in your _____ _____?

P: Not really, but I've lost some weight in the last _____ or _____ months.

D: Have you noticed anything else besides the _____ _____?

P: Well, I seem to need to go to the _____ much more often than I used to, especially at night.

D: How often do you go to the bathroom at night?

P: Three or four times. I feel very _____, so I drink a lot. That may be why.

D: Do you have any pain or discomfort in your _____?

P: Not really, but I sometime have some slight back pain. It comes and goes when I'm lying in bed.

7. Diabetes mellitus 97

Clinical exercises

1. **What disease is the patient most likely to have?**

    a   Anemia

    b   Nephritis

    c   Thyroiditis

    d   Renal stone

    e   Pancreatic cancer

2. **Which examination will be the most useful in diagnosing the above disease?**

    a   ECG

    b   Chest X-ray

    c   Urine analysis

    d   Abdominal X-ray

    e   Abdominal ultrasound exam

3. **Which of the following tests is the most useful for diagnosing diabetes mellitus?**

    a   HbA1c

    b   Urinary glucose

    c   Blood glucose level

    d   Immunoreactive insulin

    e   Oral glucose tolerance test

4. **Which of the following conditions is commonly found in patients with type 1 diabetes mellitus?**

    a   Obesity

    b   Insulin resistance

    c   Twin concurrence

    d   Response to sulfonylurea

    e   Impaired insulin secretion

Check your answers.

Doctor-patient conversation

A 59-year-old male patient visits a specialist for advice concerning the results of a recent health check-up.

D : Good morning. What's brought you here today?

P : Well, doctor, I had a regular check-up last week, and there seems to be a problem with my **hemoglobin level**.

D : Have you ever been diagnosed with[1] **anemia**?

P : No, never. But my doctor once said my blood was denser than normal. He said it was probably because I **smoke**.

D : I see. (*He looks at the results.*) Actually, according to these results, it's your HbA1c level that's high, not the hemoglobin level. And your **fasting** blood glucose is **145** mg/dL. That's above normal.

P : What's the difference between HbA1c and hemoglobin?

D : Well, the HbA1c level indicates the glucose level in the blood,[2] so it's used to diagnose **diabetes mellitus**.

P : Diabetes? I've never been diagnosed with diabetes.

D : (*He checks the past data.*) Well, your HbA1c level was around five in past years. Have there been any changes in your **lifestyle** since last year? Especially in your **daily diet**?

P : Not really, but I've lost some weight in the last **3** or **4** months.

D : Have you noticed anything else besides[3] the **weight loss**?

P : Well, I seem to need to go to the **bathroom** much more often than I used to, especially at night.

D : How often do you go to the bathroom at night?

be diagnosed with ...
…と診断される

mg/dL 読み方は
milligrams per
deciliter

HbA1c
読み方は
h-b-a-one-c

7. Diabetes mellitus　99

P : Three or four times. I feel very **thirsty**, so I drink a lot. That may be why.

D : Do you have any pain or discomfort in your **abdomen**?

P : Not really, but I sometime have some slight back pain. It comes and goes when I'm lying in bed.

Exercises

- **Find out about the HbA1c test and explain its importance for patients with diabetes. Use the information below to help you.**

HbA1cテストは，糖化ヘモグロビンテストのことですが，糖尿病のコントロール状況をみる大切な検査です。糖化ヘモグロビンは，身体中に酸素を運ぶ赤血球内のヘモグロビンが，血液中の糖と結合して糖化すると増えていきます。

糖化ヘモグロビンを測定することで，医師は，8〜12週にわたる平均的な血糖値がどれほどだったのかを知ることができます。

糖尿病の患者さんにとって，この検査は重要です。なぜならHbA1cの値が高ければ高いほど糖尿病関連の合併症を発症する危険性があるからです。

Note how the following common phrases are used in medical interviews.

❶ Have you ever been diagnosed with ...?（…と診断されたことはありますか。）

- diagnose は動詞で，本来は人を目的語にはしないとされてきたが，近年は慣用的に be diagnosed with ... も許容されつつある。

1）医師が病気を○○と診断する

The doctor **diagnosed** the illness **as** influenza.

（医師はその病気をインフルエンザと診断した。）

2）患者さんが○○と診断される

His condition **was diagnosed as** some type of blood disorder.

（彼の症状はなんらかの血液疾患と診断された。）

The patient **was diagnosed with** diabetes.（患者は糖尿病と診断された。）

- diagnose の名詞形は diagnosis，複数形は diagnoses。

The patient **was given a diagnosis of** bronchial pneumonia.

（患者は気管支肺炎と診断された。）

❷ The HbA1c level indicates the glucose level in the blood.

（HbA1c 値は血糖値［血液中のグルコース値］を反映します。）

患者さんにテストや検査の内容を説明するときに使う表現。

A viral test **is done to** find infections.

（ウイルス検査は感染をみつけるために行います。）

A throat culture **is a test used to find** germs that can cause infections.

（咽頭培養は，感染を起こしている細菌をみつけるための検査です。）

Your doctor will use a test called spirometry **to check how** your lungs are working.

（医師は，あなたの肺がどのように機能しているかを探るために，肺活量測定法とよばれる検査をします。）

❸ Have you noticed anything else besides ...?

（…のほかに気づいたことはありますか。）

診察において，できるだけ多くの症状を引き出すときに使われる定型表現。

Do you have any other symptoms that are worrying you besides ...?

（…のほかにお困りの症状はありますか。）

7. Diabetes mellitus　101

IV. Further Study

Search for information about the diagnosis, classification, treatments and prevention of diabetes mellitus through the Internet and academic papers. Also briefly explain the obtained information in simple English, the way you would do when talking to a patient.

A. Criteria for diagnosing of diabetes mellitus

B. Definition of gestational diabetes

C. Metabolic surgery as a treatment of diabetes mellitus

D. Explain the mechanisms of the following anti-diabetic drugs:
   α - glucosidase inhibitors ; DPP-4 inhibitors (dipeptidyl peptidase IV inhibitors) ; SGLT2 (sodium glucose co-transporter) inhibitors

E. How can diabetes mellitus be prevented?

8. Chronic kidney disease

慢性腎臓病 (chronic kidney disease, CKD) は慢性に経過する腎臓病の総合的な疾患概念で，糖尿病性腎症，慢性糸球体腎炎，高血圧性腎障害などの疾患概念とは別に，その腎機能 (糸球体濾過量 glomerular filtration rate, GFR) の低下と腎障害の存在から定義し分類したものです。CKDは進行すると末期慢性腎不全に至り腎代替療法が必要となるのみならず，心血管疾患 (cardiovascular disease, CVD) の危険因子となることが知られています。

Pre-reading activities

Do the following exercise before class.

1. What does the term "chronic" mean when used to describe medical conditions?

2. What is the opposite of "chronic" in this sense?

3. Define "glomerular filtration rate."

4. What kind of people have a high risk of developing CKD?

5. What are the key ways to protect against CKD progression?

6. What is ESRD?

I. Reading

Read the following passage and answer the questions that follow it.

What is chronic kidney disease?

Chronic kidney disease (CKD) is a not only a cause of end-stage renal disease (ESRD) which requires renal replacement therapy such as hemodialysis, peritoneal dialysis, and renal transplantation, but also a risk factor for cardiovascular disease (CVD).

CKD is usually a progressive disease, although people who have CKD are often unaware of their disease. CKD is without any specific symptom in its early stages.

Diabetes mellitus, hypertension, and glomerular nephritis are common causes of CKD.

Definition of chronic kidney disease

CKD is defined as abnormalities of kidney structure or function persistent for over 3 months, including evidence of kidney damage such as persistent proteinuria defined as 0.15 g/gCr (albuminuria defined as ≥30 mg/gCr [1]) for 3 months and/or reduction of kidney function defined as a GFR (glomerular filtration rate) <60 mL/min/1.73 m^2 [2] for 3 months.

GFR can be estimated from calibrated serum creatinine and from estimating equations, such as the Modification of Diet in Renal Disease (MDRD) study equation, which is called estimated GFR (eGFR). The following equations of eGFR were developed for Japanese patients:

eGFR (mL/min/1.73 m^2) =

$194 \times$ serum creatinine$^{(-1.094)} \times$ age$^{(-0.287)}$ (male) [3]

$194 \times$ serum creatinine$^{(-1.094)} \times$ age$^{(-0.287)} \times 0.739$ (female)

CKD was formerly classified into five stages in the first guideline based on the eGFR; the new classification is based on the cause (diabetes mellitus or other diseases), eGFR (G1, G2, G3a, G3b, G4, G5), and urinary albumin (A1, A2, A3).

---

abnormality 異常

persistent 持続する

proteinuria 蛋白尿

calibrate 補正する

estimating equation 推算式

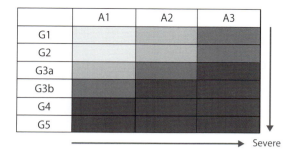

Figure 1. Staging of chronic kidney disease.
Risks of death, end-stage renal failure and death by cardiovascular disease will increase with the increasing darkness in each column.

Kidney failure (renal failure) is usually defined as an eGFR <15 mL/min/1.73 m². ❶

How to detect chronic kidney disease

It is very important to detect CKD at an early stage, before the symptoms of the renal failure appear. Treatment may slow the progression rate, which reduces the number of patients who will need renal replacement therapy.

The key issues in managing CKD are
- ensuring the etiology is correct
- implementing appropriate therapy
- monitoring the patient
- screening for CKD complications
- educating the patient.

Not all patients with decreased eGFR or low-grade albuminuria will progress to kidney failure. It is important to identify and slow progression among patients at high risk for progressive disease. In general, disease progression is often associated with high levels of albuminuria, progressive decrease in eGFR, and poorly controlled blood pressure.

To detect CKD, eGFR, urine albumin-to-creatinine ratio (UACR), and urine protein can be checked during a regular medical checkup or by one's primary care doctor.

implement 実施する

screen 検査する

urine protein 尿蛋白

medical checkup 健康診断

Keys to managing chronic kidney disease

The keys to slowing progression of CKD are to:

- control blood pressure (with angiotensin-converting enzyme inhibitors, angiotensin receptor blockers)
- reduce albuminuria
- manage diabetes
- avoid acute kidney injury.

As eGFR declines, complications occur more commonly and are more severe. These may include:

- cardiovascular disease (CVD) and dyslipidemia
- anemia due to impaired erythropoiesis and low iron stores
- mineral imbalances and bone disorders (calcium, phosphorus, and vitamin D)
- hyperkalemia
- metabolic acidosis
- malnutrition (low serum albumin)
- fluid and salt retention, often associated with accelerated hypertension.

iron store 鉄貯蔵

phosphorus リン

retention
〔本来排出されるべき
分泌物の〕滞留
accelerated
加速性の，急激な

Comprehension questions

1. **What are the common causes of CKD?**

2. **How is CKD classified?**

3. **List the complications of CKD.**

II. Vocabulary

☐ acute kidney injury	急性腎障害
☐ albuminuria	アルブミン尿
☐ angiotensin receptor blocker (ARB)	アンジオテンシン受容体拮抗薬
☐ angiotensin-converting enzyme (ACE) inhibitor	アンジオテンシン変換酵素阻害薬
☐ chronic kidney disease (CKD)	慢性腎臓病
☐ end-stage renal disease (ESRD)	末期腎不全《腎機能が低下して残腎機能が30%以下になった場合を「腎不全」とよぶ。さらに腎機能が10%以下まで低下した状態を末期腎不全とよぶ。》
☐ estimated GFR (eGFR)	推算糸球体濾過量
☐ etiology	病因論
☐ glomerular filtration rate (GFR)	糸球体濾過量
☐ glomerular nephritis	糸球体腎炎
☐ hemodialysis	血液透析療法
☐ hyperkalemia	高カリウム血症
☐ impaired erythropoiesis	赤血球生成能力の低下
☐ kidney failure, renal failure	腎不全
☐ malnutrition	栄養不良
☐ metabolic acidosis	代謝性アシドーシス
☐ mineral imbalance	電解質異常
☐ peritoneal dialysis	腹膜透析療法
☐ progressive disease	進行性疾患
☐ renal replacement therapy	腎代替療法《腎機能が低下し，生命維持が困難になったときには，腎臓の働きの代わりを担う治療が必要となる。そのような治療を「腎代替療法」とよび，血液透析療法，腹膜透析療法，腎移植の3つの方法をまとめて指す。》
☐ renal transplantation	腎移植
☐ serum creatinine	血清クレアチニン
☐ the Modification of Diet in Renal Disease (MDRD)	MDRD式《推算糸球体濾過率の計算式の一つ》

III. Medical communication

Listen to the recording of the following description of CKD and fill in the blanks. Then do the exercises that follow.

The kidneys are two bean-shaped organs, each one about the size of a fist. Your kidneys _____ wastes and excess water out of your blood and make _____.

In patients with chronic kidney disease (CKD), the kidneys are damaged and cannot filter blood the way they should. The disease is called "_____" because the damage to the kidneys happens slowly over a long period of time.

To keep your body working properly, the kidneys balance the salts and _____—such as calcium, _____, sodium, and _____—that circulate in the blood. Your kidneys also make _____ that help control _____ _____, make red blood cells, and keep your bones strong.

Kidney disease often gets worse over time and may lead to _____ _____. If your kidneys fail, you will need _____ or a _____ _____ to maintain your health.

You are at _____ for kidney disease if you have _____, high blood pressure, heart disease, or a family history of kidney failure.

Your chances of having kidney disease increase with age. The longer you have had diabetes, high blood pressure or _____ _____, the more likely it is that you will develop kidney disease.

CKD is _____ among adults in the United States. More than _____ _____ American adults may have CKD. African Americans, _____, and American Indians tend to have a greater risk of CKD, mainly because they have higher rates of diabetes and high blood pressure. Scientists are studying other possible reasons for the increased risk.

Testing is the only way to find out if you have kidney disease. Get checked if you have diabetes, high blood pressure, heart disease, or a family history of kidney failure. The sooner you know you have kidney disease, the sooner you can get treatment.

108

Clinical exercises

1. **The following chart shows the prognosis of CKD by GFR and albuminuria category. What does the range from A1 to A3 indicate?**

   a eGFR

   b Age

   c Urine protein

   d BMI

   e Blood pressure

	A1	A2	A3
G1			
G2			
G3a			
G3b			
G4			
G5			

   → Severe

2. **Which of the following is a common sign of acute renal transplant rejection?**

   a Thrombocytopenia

   b An enlarged renal graft

   c Increased blood flow to the renal graft

   d An episode of rejection within six hours

   e Effect of class I antigen of the donor on that of the recipient

3. **Which result indicates acute kidney failure requiring dialysis?**

   a Serum uric acid 10mg/dL

   b Blood urea nitrogen 38mg/dL

   c Serum potassium 7.0mEq/L

   d Arterial blood HCO_3^- 20mgEq/L

   e Serum creatinine 1.8mg/dL

(Translation of the National Examination for Medical Practitioners 110I14, 110E1, 110E5)

Check your answers.

The kidneys are two bean-shaped organs, each one about the size of a fist. Your kidneys **filter** wastes and excess water out of your blood and make **urine**.

fist 握りこぶし

In patients with chronic kidney disease (CKD), the kidneys are damaged and cannot filter blood the way they should. The disease is called "**chronic**" because the damage to the kidneys happens slowly over a long period of time.

To keep your body working properly, the kidneys balance the salts and **minerals**—such as calcium, **phosphorus**, sodium, and **potassium**—that circulate in the blood. Your kidneys also make **hormones** that help control **blood pressure**, make red blood cells, and keep your bones strong.

mineral ミネラル
calcium カルシウム
sodium ナトリウム
potassium カリウム

Kidney disease often gets worse over time and may lead to **kidney failure**. If your kidneys fail, you will need **dialysis** or a **kidney transplant** to maintain your health.

You are at **risk** for kidney disease if you have [4] **diabetes**, high blood pressure, heart disease, or a family history of kidney failure.

Your chances of having kidney disease increase with age. The longer you have had diabetes, high blood pressure or **heart disease**, the more likely it is that you will develop kidney disease.

CKD is **common** among adults in the United States. More than **20 million** American adults may have CKD. African Americans, **Hispanics**, and American Indians tend to have a greater risk of CKD, [4] mainly because they have higher rates of diabetes and high blood pressure. Scientists are studying other possible reasons for the increased risk.

Testing is the only way to find out if you have kidney disease. Get checked if you have diabetes, high blood pressure, heart disease, or a family history of kidney failure. The sooner you know you have kidney disease, the sooner you can get treatment.[5]

Exercises

- **Write a case report on the following patient and present it in the class.**

40歳，男性。長期にわたり高血圧症と糖尿病に罹患。嘔気，嘔吐と下肢に浮腫あり。体重は80kg。血圧は180/120。24時間の蓄尿検査の結果，尿量は850 mL, 尿蛋白は600 mg/dL, 尿クレアチニンは180 mg/dLである。

Note how the following common phrases are used in case reports.

❶ albuminuria ≥30mg/gCr, GFR <60 mL/min/1.73 m^2,
eGFR <15 mL/min/1.73 m^2

（アルブミン尿は30mg/gCr以上，GFRは60mL/分/1.73m²未満，eGFRは15mL/分/1.73m²未満）

検査の基準を示す不等号の読み方はそれぞれ下記のとおり。

A > B　（AはB超）：A is greater than B

A ≥ B　（AはB以上）：A is greater than or equal to B

A < B　（AはB未満）：A is less than B

A ≤ B　（AはB以下）：A is less than or equal to B

ただし，検査結果の数値に問題があることを患者さんに伝える場合には，is (a little/rather) high/lowなどの表現を用いて伝える。

- According to the test results, your GFR **is rather low**.

（検査によると，GFRがかなり減少しています。）

- The test results indicate that the protein level in your urine **is a little high**.

（検査結果によると，尿蛋白が少し高いです。）

❷ **60 mL/min/1.73 m^2, 30 mg/gCr**

口頭では単位を省くことが多いが，読むときはそれぞれ下記の通り。

- 60 mL/min/1.73 m^2：sixty **milliliters per minute per** one point seven three **square meter**
- 30 mg/gCr：thirty **milligrams per gram creatinine**

❸ eGFR (mL/min/1.73 m^2) = **194 × serum creatinine $^{(-1.094)}$ × age $^{(-0.287)}$**

数式を口頭で発表する場合には，下記の通り。

- eGFR **equals** one hundred ninety-four **multiplied by** serum creatinine **to the power of** minus one point zero nine four **multiplied by** age **to the power of** minus zero point two eight seven.

❹ You **are at risk for** kidney disease if you have ....

African Americans tend to **have a greater risk of** CKD.

危険因子を説明する際によく使われる表現。be at risk for ... もしくは have a risk of ... で「…の危険性がある」の意味。

❺ **The sooner** you know you have kidney disease, **the sooner** you can get

treatment. （早く…に気づけば気づくほど，早く〜できる。）

患者さんに手術や治療を勧める場合によく使われる表現。

- **The longer** you have had diabetes, high blood pressure or heart disease,
the more likely it is that you will develop kidney disease.

（長く…すればするほど，ますます〜の可能性が高くなる。）

112

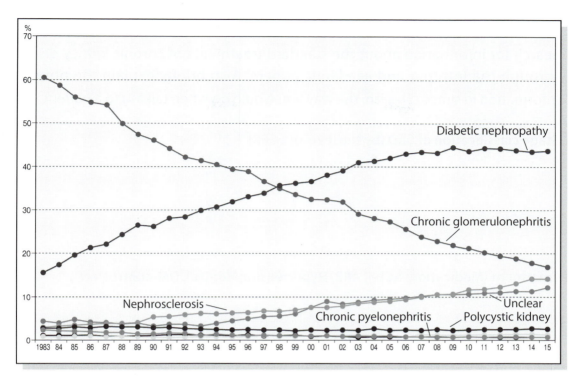

Figure 1. Rates of new patients with different primary diseases started on dialysis in Japan (1983–2015).

(Adapted from "An overview of regular dialysis treatment in Japan as of Dec. 31, 2015" by Japanese Society for Dialysis Therapy <http://docs.jsdt.or.jp/overview/pdf2016/2015all.pdf>)

Medical Background

Modification of Diet in Renal Disease (MDRD)

　腎機能を評価するにあたっては，推定糸球体濾過量（estimated glomerular filtration rate, eGFR）やクレアチニンクリアランス（creatinine clearance, Ccr）が用いられます。Ccrは血清クレアチニン値（serum creatinine, Scr）を用いて下記の計算式で求めます。

　　Ccr =（140 − age）x weight /（72 x Scr）　＊女性の場合は左式 x 0.85

　Ccrよりさらに正確な値を求めるための計算式として考案されたのがMDRD式で，1999年の発表後に修正が加えられ，現在は下記のMDRD175が世界的に用いられています。

　　eGFR [mL/min/1.73m^2] = 175 x Scr$^{-1.154}$ x age$^{-0.203}$　＊女性の場合は左式 x 0.742

　この式は母集団が白人のため，日本人にそのまま当てはめると誤った値となる可能性があるため，日本腎臓学会が2009年に日本人向けの推算式を発表しました。

　　eGFR [mL/min/1.73m^2] = 194 x Scr$^{-1.094}$ x age$^{-0.287}$　＊女性の場合は左式 x 0.739

本項もこの式を本文で取り上げています。

IV. Further Study

Search for information about the standard treatments of chronic kidney disease, through the Internet and academic papers. Also briefly explain the obtained information in simple English, the way you would do when talking to a patient.

A. Stage classification of CKD (by the level of eGFR)

B. Treatment (Medication: ACE-I, ARB, Hypertension-control, DM-control, etc.)

C. Treatment (Nutrition: sodium restriction, protein restriction, potassium restriction, etc.)

D. Complications (Metabolic acidosis, hyperkalemia, anemia, secondary hyperparathyroidism, etc.)

E. Renal replacement therapy (hemodialysis, peritoneal dialysis, renal transplantation)

9. Malignant lymphoma

　悪性リンパ腫 (malignant lymphoma) は，リンパ球の分化過程で生じた腫瘍形成性腫瘍の総称です。特徴は，①全身あらゆるリンパ節およびリンパ節外の組織に発生して，きわめて多彩な症状を呈する点，②診断は病理組織診断によってなされ，病理組織分類が多様である点，③化学療法・放射線療法に対する感受性が高く，基本的には延命ではなくて治癒を目指した治療を求められる点です。

Pre-reading activities

Do the following exercise before class.

1. Which lymph nodes are commonly enlarged in patients with malignant lymphoma?

2. How is malignant lymphoma diagnosed?

3. What are the two major types of malignant lymphoma?
   Which is more common?

4. What is the standard chemotherapy used for diffuse large B-cell lymphoma?

5. What factors determine the prognosis of patients with aggressive lymphoma?

9. Malignant lymphoma　115

I. Reading

Read the following passages and answer the questions that follow them.

Passage 1

Lymphoma is a cancer of lymphocytes that develops not only in the lymph nodes but also in various extranodal lymphoid tissues. Therefore, in addition to causing enlargement of lymph nodes (e.g. cervical, axillary, and inguinal lymph nodes), it also causes extremely diverse clinical manifestations, including skin rash, respiratory failure, gastrointestinal obstruction, cardiac tamponade, paralyses, and urinary obstruction.

The annual incidence of malignant lymphoma in Japan has been increasing: it was 5.5 per 100,000 people in 1985, 8.9 in 1995, and 13.3 in 2005. The male to female ratio is approximately 3:2, and the disease most commonly affects patients aged 65 to 74 years.

Histologically, malignant lymphoma is classified as Hodgkin lymphoma (accounting for 4% to 5% of cases in Japan) or non-Hodgkin lymphoma. The former is characterized by the presence of Reed Sternberg cells, while the latter is divided into B-cell type (65%-70%) and T/NK cell type (25%-30%); both are further categorized into more than 20 subtypes on the basis of the molecular features of the lymphoma cells, such as cell-surface phenotypes and chromosomal abnormalities. The incidence of some subtypes of lymphoma differs according to geographic location. In Western countries, for example, the incidence of Hodgkin lymphoma is relatively high, while that of T/NK cell lymphoma is relatively low.

Although the etiology of most types of lymphoma is still unknown, some types are known to be associated with certain viruses. Adult T-cell leukemia/lymphoma, which is prevalent in Japan and in the Caribbean, is causally linked to human T-cell leukemia virus type 1 (HTLV-1). Extranodal nasal type NK/T-cell lymphoma, which is prevalent in Southern Asia, Japan and parts of Latin America, is almost always associated

extranodal lymphoid tissue
節外性リンパ組織

respiratory failure
呼吸不全

gastrointestinal obstruction
胃腸管閉塞

cardiac tamponade
心タンポナーデ

urinary obstruction
尿路閉塞

annual incidence
年間発生率

chromosomal abnormality
染色体異常

with Epstein-Barr virus (EBV).

An excisional biopsy (rather than fine-needle aspiration) is necessary for the histological diagnosis of malignant lymphoma. Since various diseases cause lymphadenopathy, doctors need to decide whether to perform biopsies for patients with lymphadenopathy. Differential diagnoses include infectious diseases such as infectious mononucleosis, non-infectious inflammation (caused, for example, by sarcoidosis or autoimmune diseases, such as SLE), and metastases of solid tumors (as, for example, in gastric cancer). When the patient is young (particularly less than 30 years old) or the lymph nodes show marked inflammatory tendencies, such as tenderness, there is little likelihood of lymphoma. However, when the lymph nodes are large and growing rapidly, or the serum lactate dehydrogenase (LDH) is elevated, there is a significant likelihood of lymphoma.

excisional biopsy
摘出生検，切除生検

fine-needle aspiration
細針吸引生検《fine-needle aspirateのほうが容易（外来受診時にその場で可能）で，excisional biopsyは出血等のリスクが高く（しばしば）入院を要する。しかしながら，前者は癌（例えば胃癌患者の頸部リンパ節が「転移」かどうかの判定）には有用かつ十分だが，リンパ腫の病型診断には不十分》

mononucleosis
単核細胞症

serum lactate dehydrogenase (LDH)
血清乳酸脱水素酵素

Comprehension questions 1

1. **What are the symptoms of lymphoma? Give some examples.**

2. **According to the passage, which gender and age groups are at high risk for lymphoma?**

3. **Which subtype of lymphoma is less prevalent in Japan than in Western countries?**

4. **What diagnostic possibilities should be considered for patients with lymphadenopathy?**

Passage 2

After a diagnosis of lymphoma is made, computed tomography (CT) scans, positron emission tomography (PET) scans, and bone marrow examinations are used to evaluate the extent of the disease according to the Ann Arbor staging system. Stage I is defined as the involvement of a single lymph node, stage II as the involvement of two or more lymph nodes on the same side of the diaphragm, stage III as two or more on both sides of the diaphragm, and stage IV is defined as a disseminated disease involving, for example, the bone marrow. Fever (>38°C), night sweats, and weight loss (>10% of body weight in the 6 months preceding admission) are defined as B symptoms.

To predict the prognosis of patients with aggressive lymphoma, a clinical prognostic model known as the International Prognostic Index (IPI) is widely used; this index categorizes the patients into risk groups. There are five factors that indicate an adverse prognosis: age over 60 years, Ann Arbor stage III or IV, elevated serum lactate dehydrogenase, Eastern Cooperative Oncology Group (ECOG) performance status of 2 or greater, and involvement of more than one extranodal site.

Malignant lymphoma is one of the most sensitive tumors to chemotherapy and radiotherapy. For diffuse large B-cell lymphoma, which is the most common type of B-cell lymphoma, 6 to 8 cycles of R-CHOP therapy, consisting of cyclophosphamide, doxorubicin (Hydroxydaunomycin®), vincristine (Oncovin®), and prednisone plus rituximab, has been established as the standard chemotherapy, achieving a 5-year overall survival rate of 60% to 70%. Patients with Ann Arbor stage I or II can be effectively treated with 3 to 4 cycles of R-CHOP therapy, followed by involved field radiotherapy. If patients relapse, salvage chemotherapy with a combination of various agents is performed, and if patients are chemotherapy-sensitive, autologous stem cell transplantation leads to long-term

disseminated
播種性の

relapse 再発する
salvage
chemotherapy
救済化学療法
autologous
stem cell
transplantation
自家幹細胞移植

disease-free survival in up to 40% of them. Allogeneic stem cell transplantation is also indicated in some cases.

allogeneic
同種の《autologousの
対比として用いられる》

Comprehension questions 2

1. If a patient had two lymph nodes on the same side of the diaphragm, a 10% weight loss over 6 months and occasional fever, what would the staging evaluation be?

2. What therapy would be effective for patients with early stage malignant lymphoma?

3. What are the factors that indicate a poor prognosis in patients with aggressive lymphoma?

4. If patients with diffuse large B-cell lymphoma relapse after the initial chemotherapy, and if their disease is still responsive to chemotherapy, what would be the most likely treatment?

9. Malignant lymphoma 119

II. Vocabulary

Incidence	**発生率，発病率**
Etiology	**病因**
☐ tumor suppressor gene	癌抑制遺伝子
☐ Epstein-Barr virus (EB virus)	エプスタイン・バー（EB）ウイルス
☐ human T-cell leukemia virus 1 (HTLV-1)	ヒトT細胞白血病ウイルス
☐ human immunodeficiency virus (HIV)	ヒト免疫不全ウイルス
Symptoms	**症状**
☐ lymphadenopathy	リンパ節症
☐ B symptoms	B症状
☐ night sweats	盗汗，寝汗
☐ hepatomegaly	肝腫大
☐ splenomegaly	脾腫
☐ Performance Status	パフォーマンスステータス
Diagnosis	**診断**
☐ lymph node biopsy	リンパ節生検
☐ morphology	形態学
☐ immunophenotype	免疫表現型
☐ cytogenetics	細胞遺伝学
☐ involvement	浸潤
Examination	**検査**
☐ lactate dehydrogenase (LDH)	乳酸脱水素酵素
☐ soluble interleukin-2 receptor (sIL-2R)	可溶性インターロイキン2受容体
☐ positron emission tomography (PET)	陽電子放射断層撮影〔法〕
☐ bone marrow biopsy	骨髄生検
WHO classification	**WHO分類**
☐ Hodgkin lymphoma (HL)	ホジキンリンパ腫

☐ Reed-Sternberg cell	リード・スタンバーグ細胞
☐ non-Hodgkin lymphoma (NHL)	非ホジキンリンパ腫
☐ diffuse large B cell lymphoma	びまん性大細胞型B細胞性リンパ腫
☐ follicular lymphoma	濾胞性リンパ腫
☐ Burkitt lymphoma	バーキットリンパ腫
☐ adult T cell leukemia-lymphoma	成人T細胞性白血病/リンパ腫
☐ chronic lymphocytic leukemia/small lymphocytic lymphoma	慢性リンパ性白血病／小リンパ球性リンパ腫
☐ splenic marginal zone lymphoma	脾辺縁帯リンパ腫
☐ indolent	インドレント（緩慢性）
☐ aggressive	アグレッシブ（進行性）

Prognosis 予後

☐ International Prognostic Index (IPI)	国際予後指数

Treatment 治療

☐ R-CHOP therapy	R-CHOP療法
☐ radiation therapy	放射線治療
☐ stem cell transplant	幹細胞移植
☐ autologous peripheral blood stem cell transplantation	自家末梢血幹細胞移植

Evaluation 評価

☐ Complete Response (CR)	完全奏効，著効
☐ Complete Response/ unconfirmed (CRu)	不確定完全奏効
☐ Partial Response (PR)	部分奏効，有効
☐ Stable Disease (SD)	安定
☐ Progressive Disease (PD)	進行
☐ Relapsed Disease (RD)	再発

III. Medical communication

Listen to the recording of the following case report and fill in the blanks. Then answer the questions that follow.

Case report

A 24-year-old man presented to the hospital complaining of fever and a painless mass in the neck. He had noticed the mass in the left side of his neck a month before his visit and during that time he had occasionally had fever of 37.0°C to 38.0°C. The mass has been getting a little larger. He has had no significant _____ illnesses and does not drink alcohol.

On examination, he was alert and awake. His temperature was 37.8°C. There were two non-tender smooth lymph nodes of 2 cm in diameter on the left side of his neck and the _____ clavicle, an axillary lymph node of 2 cm in diameter on each side, and one of 1.5 cm in diameter in the right _____ area. Enlargement of the right tonsil was noticed. Lungs were clear to auscultation bilaterally. His abdomen was flat and soft and non-distended, and his liver and _____ were not palpable.

Laboratory studies showed red blood cells 4,620,000, hemoglobin _____ g/dL, hematocrit 43%, white blood cells _____ /μL with 67% neutrophils, 8% eosinophils, 1% basophils, 4% monocytes, and 20% lymphocytes, and platelets count _____ /μL. Chemistry studies showed total protein _____ g/dL, albumin 4.2 g/dL, blood urea nitrogen (BUN) 16.0 mg/dL, creatinine 0.9 mg/dL, uric acid 7.6 mg/dL, total cholesterol 120 mg/dL, total bilirubin 0.8 mg/dL, AST _____ IU/L, ALT 32 IU/L, LD 420 and CRP 1.2 mg/dL. A chest X-ray showed a mass shadow on each hilum of the lung. The result of the

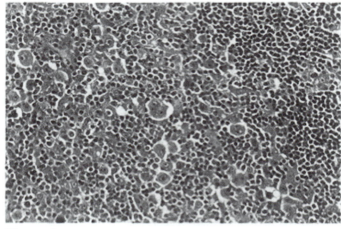

Figure 1.

cervical lymph node biopsy is shown in Figure 1.

(Translation of part of the National Examination for Medical Practitioners 102 D48)

Clinical exercises

1. **What does "His abdomen was flat and soft and non-distended" mean?**

    ----

2. **What is the most likely diagnosis for this patient?**

    a   systemic lupus erythemtosus

    b   tuberculosis

    c   adenocarcinoma

    d   Hodgkin lymphoma

    e   non-Hodgkin lymphoma

3. **Which of the following is the most appropriate treatment for this patient?**

    a   radiation therapy

    b   anti-tuberculosis therapy

    c   rituximab

    d   multiple chemotherapy

    e   glucocorticoid pulse therapy

Check your answers.

Case report

A 24-year-old man presented to the hospital complaining of fever and a painless mass in the neck. He had noticed the mass in the left side of his neck a month before his visit and during that time he had occasionally had fever of 37.0°C to 38.0°C. The mass has been getting a little larger. He has had no significant **previous** illnesses and does not drink alcohol.

On examination, he was alert[1] and awake. His temperature was 37.8°C. There were two non-tender smooth lymph nodes of 2 cm in diameter[2] on the left side of his neck and the **upper** clavicle, an axillary lymph node of 2 cm in diameter on each side, and one of 1.5 cm in diameter in the right **inguinal** area. Enlargement of the right tonsil was noticed. Lungs were clear to auscultation bilaterally.[3] His abdomen was flat and soft and non-distended, and his liver and **spleen** were not palpable.[4]

Laboratory studies showed red blood cells 4,620,000, hemoglobin **14.2** g/dL, hematocrit 43%, white blood cells **12,000**/μL[5] with 67% neutrophils, 8% eosinophils, 1% basophils, 4% monocytes, and 20% lymphocytes, and platelets count **260,000**/μL. Chemistry studies showed total protein **7.3** g/dL, albumin 4.2 g/dL, blood urea nitrogen (BUN) 16.0 mg/dL, creatinine 0.9 mg/dL, uric acid 7.6 mg/dL, total cholesterol 120 mg/dL, total bilirubin 0.8 mg/dL, AST **45** IU/L, ALT 32 IU/L, LD 420 and CRP 1.2 mg/dL. A chest X-ray showed a mass shadow on each hilum of the lung. The result of the cervical lymph node biopsy is shown in Figure 1.

---

complain of
[symptoms]
〔症状を〕訴える

alert and awake
〔意識が〕清明である

non-tender
圧痛のない

non-distended
腹部膨満なし

neutrophil 好中球
eosinophil 好酸球
basophil 好塩基球
monocyte 単球
platelet 血小板

hilum
門《神経と脈管が出入りする器官の部分》

Note how the following common terms and phrases are used in case reports.

❶ he was alert（意識は清明）

診察の際の患者の general appearance（全身状態）を述べる表現。そのほかに,

unconscious（意識消失）,

anxious（不安状態）,

restless（落ち着きのない）,

in acute distress（急迫状態にある：すぐに処置が必要なくらいぐったりしている）,

in mild distress（少し元気がない, 調子が悪そう）,

cooperative（協力的な）

などがあるが, 調子が悪そうにみえない場合には **He (she) appeared well.** のように述べる。

❷ ... cm in diameter（直径… cm）

The pupils are 3.0 **mm in diameter**, equal, and react to light and accommodation.

（瞳孔径は両側とも3mm, 対光反射および輻輳反射正常。）

❸ clear to auscultation bilaterally（異常呼吸音なし）

聴診で左右の肺に異常音がないときに述べる。

❹ (not) palpable（触知する（しない））

No intraluminal masses were **palpable**.

（管腔内腫瘤は触知しない。）

He had tender **palpable** lymphadenopathy in the right inguinal area.

（左鼠径部に圧痛を伴うリンパ節腫脹を触知した。）

❺ 検査結果の単位の読み方

dL: deciliter（デシリットル＝10分の1リットル）

μL: microliter（マイクロリットル＝100万分の1リットル）

9. Malignant lymphoma　125

Exercises

- **Write the case report of the following patient and make a presentation in the class.**

33歳，女性。1週間前より乾性咳嗽を自覚し，呼吸困難を主訴に来院した。身体診察上，リンパ節腫脹を認めず，肝臓脾臓を触知しなかった。胸部CT検査にて前縦隔に巨大な腫瘤を認め，生検にて縦隔原発大細胞型B細胞性リンパ腫と診断された。R-CHOP療法にて完全寛解が得られたが，すぐ再発した。救援療法後，自家末梢血幹細胞移植が行われ，完全寛解が得られ，10年以上維持されている。

IV. Further Study

Search for information about lymphoma through the Internet and academic papers. Also briefly explain the obtained information in simple English, the way you would do when talking to a patient.

A. Etiology of lymphoma

B. AIDS-related lymphoma

C. Recent advances in the treatment of adult T-cell leukemia-lymphoma

D. Recent approaches in the treatment of Hodgkin lymphoma

10. Infective endocarditis

　感染性心内膜炎（infective endocarditis）は血中に入ってきた細菌が心臓の弁膜に感染することにより起きる全身感染症です。発症初期は発熱や全身倦怠感など，非特異的症状が主体であり，進行すると弁膜から菌が播種された臓器固有の症状が出現します。抗菌化学療法が治療の主体となりますが，人工弁置換術が必要となる場合もあります。早期に正確に診断することが最も重要です。

Pre-reading activities

Do the following exercise before class.

1. What is the definition of "infectious diseases"?

2. Describe the differences between endocarditis and pericarditis.

3. How is infective endocarditis (IE) classified on the basis of valve types?

4. What are the main microorganisms responsible for IE?

5. What are the signs and symptoms of IE?

6. Explain the treatment options for IE.

7. What are the risk factors for developing IE?

10. Infective endocarditis　129

I. Reading

Read the following passage and answer the questions that follow it.

Definition and classification

Infective endocarditis (IE) is an endovascular infection, usually caused by bacteria, of the endocardium and cardiac valves. Because the heart functions as a pump in the circulatory system, the infectious organism causing IE is disseminated throughout the body to other organ systems.

In patients with IE, either natural or prosthetic valves can be infected. Natural valves are previously healthy or congenitally impaired valves, and prosthetic valves are artificial ones that have been surgically implanted to replace impaired natural valves.

Pathogenesis and microbiology

Staphylococci and streptococci are the leading pathogens in IE. Community-acquired IE often occurs when oral streptococci enter the bloodstream through dental procedures, such as scaling or extraction, and colonize the cardiac valves. In hospitalized patients, catheter-related blood stream infections caused by staphylococci are the leading causes of healthcare-associated or nosocomial IE. In particular, infections caused by methicillin-resistant *Staphylococcus aureus* pose a critical risk to patients.

Signs and symptoms

In its early stage, IE is often overlooked or misdiagnosed as a cold or viral infection due to its systemic symptoms, such as low-grade fever and malaise. Though oral antibiotics commonly prescribed in outpatient settings may temporarily relieve the patients' symptoms, these symptoms recur after termination of short-course treatment; IE requires treatment with intravenous administration of a combined antimicrobial regimen for at least 2 to 4 weeks. Repetition of this oral antimicrobial therapy over a prolonged period of time can cause valve vegetation and regurgitation, which can eventually lead to congestive heart failure. It is not until patients develop cardiac symptoms (e.g. dyspnea on exertion) that physicians start to recognize the seriousness of their patients' conditions.

Clinical manifestations and complications of IE resulting from microvascular impairment or emboli are variable; they include Osler's nodes on the palms and soles, Roth spots on the retina, and infarction of the kidney or spleen. IE often results in devastating conditions such as brain infarction, which are life-threatening if left untreated.

Diagnosis

The two major criteria for a definitive diagnosis of IE are: 1) positive blood cultures for bacteria strongly associated with IE, and 2) valve regurgitation or vegetation found on transthoracic or transesophageal echocardiography. Multiple blood cultures are strongly recommended for patients with fever of unknown origin to detect IE early in its clinical course.

Treatment

Treatment with antimicrobial agents, which have the maximum efficacy against the infecting organisms, is the mainstay of therapy for IE. These agents are administered intravenously for 2 to 4 weeks. If a patient's condition is complicated by metastatic infection, a longer duration of therapy is needed.

In cases where valve damage is severe enough to compromise cardiac function or where a new embolic event occurs despite appropriate antibiotic therapy, surgical intervention (usually valve replacement) is indicated.

To maximize the efficacy of treatment, it is of prime importance to assemble a multidisciplinary team consisting of an infectious disease specialist, a cardiologist, and a cardiac surgeon.

Prophylaxis

Those who undergo dental procedures are at risk of developing IE, especially those with a past history of heart disease. Antibiotic prophylaxis with penicillin is recommended for high-risk patients. However, most experts now recommend maintenance of good oral, dental, and skin hygiene rather than focusing on specific subsets of patients with cardiac conditions.

Comprehension questions

1. How does IE cause infection in organ systems other than the circulatory system?

2. Why is IE easily overlooked?

3. When should valve replacement surgery be considered?

4. What kind of prophylaxis is available for IE?

II. Vocabulary

☐ acquired immunodeficiency (immune deficiency) syndrome (AIDS)	後天性免疫不全症候群，エイズ
☐ acute poliomyelitis	急性灰白髄炎
☐ bacteremia	菌血症
☐ catheter-related blood stream infection	カテーテル関連血流感染症《血管内に留置したカテーテル＝異物を媒介する菌血症》
☐ cellulitis	蜂窩織炎
☐ cephalosporin	セファロスポリン系抗菌薬
☐ cholera	コレラ
☐ community-acquired infection	市中感染症
☐ conjunctivitis	結膜炎
☐ cystitis	膀胱炎
☐ Dengue fever	デング熱
☐ diphtheria	ジフテリア
☐ disseminate	播種する《種をまいたかのように細菌などが最初に感染した場所から離脱し体全体に広がること》
☐ enterococcus, [pl.]— cocci	腸球菌
☐ epidemic	流行病，伝染病，疫病
☐ epidemic parotitis, mumps	流行性耳下腺炎，おたふくかぜ
☐ febrile	熱がある《「熱がない」はafebrile 。熱中症などの際の高体温はhyperthermia》
☐ foodborne disease	食品媒介疾患《Anisakis, Salmonella などで発症する疾患》
☐ healthcare-associated infection	医療関連感染症
☐ *Haemophilus influenzae* type b (Hib)	ヘモフィルス・インフルエンザ菌b型
☐ herpes zoster, shingles	帯状疱疹
☐ intermittent fever	間欠熱《発熱と解熱を繰り返す状態が続くこと》

10. Infective endocarditis 133

☐ leukocytosis	白血球増加症
☐ malaria	マラリア
☐ measles	麻疹
☐ methicillin-resistant *Staphylococcus aureus* (MRSA)	メチシリン耐性黄色ブドウ球菌
☐ microbiology	微生物学
☐ Middle East respiratory syndrome (MERS)	中東呼吸器症候群
☐ multidisciplinary	多専門職の《cf. multidisciplinary approach 集学的アプローチ（「チーム医療」と訳してもよい）》
☐ nosocomial	病院の中で起きる《cf. nosocomial infection 院内感染症》
☐ opportunistic infection	日和見感染症《免疫能が低下した患者における弱毒菌による感染症》
☐ orchitis, orchiditis	睾丸炎
☐ Osler's node	オスラー結節《感染性心内膜炎で指尖や足底に認められる赤紫調の有痛性あるいは無痛性の皮膚病変》
☐ otitis media	中耳炎
☐ pandemic	広域に及ぶ感染病の大流行
☐ penicillin	ペニシリン系抗菌薬
☐ pertussis, whooping cough	百日咳
☐ pleuritis	胸膜炎
☐ prophylaxis	予防
☐ pyelonephritis	腎盂腎炎
☐ Roth spot	ロス斑《血行播種された菌による網膜の末梢循環異常を表す眼底所見》
☐ rubella, German measles	風疹
☐ severe acute respiratory syndrome (SARS)	重症急性呼吸器症候群
☐ staphylococcus, [pl.]— cocci	ブドウ球菌属《*Staphylococcus aureus* 黄色ブドウ球菌》
☐ streptococcus, [pl.]— cocci	レンサ球菌属

☐ susceptibility	感受性，感染しやすさ	
☐ systemic infection, systemic infectious disease	全身感染症	
☐ tetanus, lockjaw	破傷風	
☐ tinea pedis, athlete's foot	足白癬，水虫	
☐ tuberculosis (TB)	結核	
☐ typhoid fever	腸チフス	
☐ vaccination	ワクチン接種，予防接種	
☐ varicella, chickenpox	水痘	
☐ vegetation	疣贅	

III. Medical communication

Listen to the following dialog between a resident (R) and an attending doctor (AD) and fill in the blanks. Then do the exercises that follow it.

Doctor-doctor conversation

R : resident AD : attending doctor

AD: So, please tell me about the patient.

R : The patient is a _____-year-old man who was _____ _____ a nearby clinic with fever and cardiac murmur.

AD: What are the _____ of the heart murmur?

R : Well, on _____, a murmur _____ of mitral regurgitation is heard.

AD: In that case, what infectious disease, if _____, can _____ to a serious condition?

R : I think we should check for infective _____.

AD: Right. And what tests do we need to perform immediately to make a _____ _____?

R : An _____.

AD: That's right. Have you taken blood cultures to identify the causative microorganism?

R : Yes, I've already sent 2 sets of blood cultures to the _____.

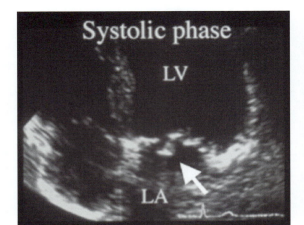 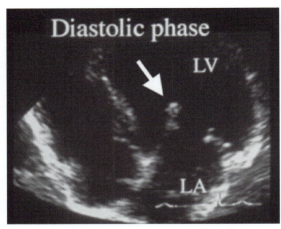

Figure 1. Mitral valve vegetation protruding toward the left ventricle during the diastolic phase (arrows).
LA: left atrium, LV: left ventricle

AD: Good. Are there any _____ to make you _____ central nervous system complications?

R : No. No _____ motor paralysis or paresthesia.

AD: Then let's go and check to see if he has any cranial nerve _____.

Clinical exercises

1. **What are likely causes of heart murmur?**

2. **What heart sounds are characteristic of IE?**

3. **What are the two major criteria for making a definitive diagnosis of IE?**

4. **What are the two methods of performing echocardiography?**

5. **What microorganisms account for the majority of cases of IE?**

6. **Why is it necessary to check the patient's central nervous system?**

7. **What treatment should be given if the patient is diagnosed with IE?**

10. Infective endocarditis 137

Check your answers.

Doctor-doctor conversation

AD : So, please tell me about the patient.

R : The patient is a **52**-year-old man who was **referred from** a nearby clinic with fever and cardiac murmur.[1]

AD : What are the **characteristics** of the heart murmur?

R : Well, on **auscultation**,[2] a murmur **suggestive** of mitral regurgitation is heard.[3]

AD : In that case, what infectious disease, if **overlooked**, can **lead** to a serious condition?[4]

R : I think we should check for[5] infective **endocarditis**.

AD : Right. And what tests do we need to perform immediately to make a **definitive diagnosis**?[6]

R : An **echocardiography**.

AD : That's right. Have you taken blood cultures to identify the **causative** microorganism?[7]

R : Yes, I've already sent 2 sets of blood cultures to the **lab**.

AD : Good. Are there any **findings** to make you **suspect**[8] central nervous system complications?

R : No. No **apparent**[9] motor paralysis or paresthesia.

AD : Then let's go and check to see if he has any cranial nerve **abnormalities**.

138

Note how the following common terms and phrases are used in case reports.

❶ The patient is a 52-year-old man who was **referred from** a nearby clinic **with** fever and cardiac murmur.

（患者は52歳，男性で，発熱と心雑音により近医から紹介されてきた。）

　患者が他の医院・病院から紹介されてきたときにはA was referred from …を用い，他の施設へ紹介するときにはrefer A to …を用いる。例文のように「…の症状で」紹介されてきたときはwith … (fever)を用い，「…する目的で」紹介されたときはfor (an evaluation of) …のような表現を用いる。紹介状はreferral letterだが，referralだけでも用いられる。

Do you have a **referral**?（紹介状はお持ちですか。）

　主治医等に短時間で患者の症状を報告するときには，重要な情報を先に述べることがある。例文ではreferred from a nearby clinicを先に述べているが，The patient is a 52-year-old man **with** fever and cardiac murmur **who was referred from** a nearby clinic. と症状を先に述べることもある（英語ではelevator speechという慣用表現があり，エレベーターに乗っている短時間に行う要を得た簡潔な報告を意味する）。例えば，既往歴や家族歴などでも鑑別に重要だと思われれば主訴より先に述べることもある。

Mrs. Jones, a 35-year-old woman **with** diabetes mellitus, **presented to** the clinic concerned about a chest pain that started 2 days ago.

　一般に主訴はchief complaint (CC)で，The patient presented to the clinic with … という表現を使う場合が多いが，近年は，患者がcomplain（文句を言う）という表現を嫌がるために，上記の例文のように **concerned about** を代わりに用いることも増えてきたという。この場合，主訴はchief concernで，同じCCの略語を用いる。

❷ **on auscultation**, …（聴診では…）

　触診はpalpation，打診はpercussion。ただしこれらは専門用語なので，患者さんに話すときはI'm going to **listen to** your lungs.や**touch, tap**のような一般用語 (lay terms)を用いる。

❸ …murmur **suggestive of** mitral regurgitation is heard.

（僧帽弁逆流を疑う心雑音を聴取します。）

確かではないが何かが疑われるときに使われる表現。… **is suspected** も使われる。

❹ What infectious disease, **if overlooked**, can lead to a serious condition?

（見落とすと重篤な結果につながる感染症は何だと思いますか。）

　徴候や病気を見落とすと，というときに使われる表現。**misdiagnose**（誤診する）や**miss the signs**（徴候を見落とす）などもよく用いられる。なお，見落としてはならない危険信号のことをwarning signやred flagともいう。

❺ We should **check for** …（…の有無を確かめるべきである。）

10. Infective endocarditis 　139

❻ **make a definitive diagnosis**（確定診断をする）

　鑑別診断は**differential diagnosis**で，会話では単に**differentials**ともいう（通常は複数形）。確定診断のために検査を行って他の病気を除外するときには**rule out**をよく用いる。

❼ **identify** the **causative** microorganism（原因微生物を特定する）

　identifyは「確定する・特定する」という意味でよく使われる。ここでは原因菌の種名を調べ確定するという意味で使われているので「原因菌を同定する」と訳す。また**determine**（判定する・見極める）のような表現も使われる。

　causativeは「原因となる」という意味でcausative allergen, causative agent, causative diseaseのように用いられる。

❽ **Are there any findings to make you suspect ...?**（…を疑う所見はありますか。）

❾ **no** apparent ...（明らかな…はありません）

　徴候がまったくないときには，apparentを抜いて**no ...**と表現することもできる。注目すべき徴候がないときには，**no ... of note**などの表現を用いる。また，患者自身が述べた症状を報告するときは，The patient **reports/states/recalls/noted**等の表現を用い，患者が否定しているときにはThe patient **reports no** ...やThe patient **denies** ...のような表現を用いる。

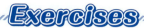

- **Role-playing: Following the example above, make a dialog between a resident and an attending doctor based on the following case report, and then role-play in pairs.**

21歳，女性。2週間前からの微熱と咳嗽で近医を受診した。マイコプラズマ肺炎（Mycoplasma pneumonia）が疑われ抗菌薬の投与を受けたが，症状が改善されなかったため当院を紹介されてきた。膿性痰（purulent sputum）の喀出はない（non-productive cough/dry cough）。

呼吸音（lung sounds/respiratory sounds）は正常。持参した胸部X線像（chest radiogram）では右肺上葉（right upper lobe）に空洞を伴う浸潤影（cavitary infiltrate）が認められた。抗菌薬の投与を受けていたが症状は改善しない。重篤な感染症としては肺結核（pulmonary tuberculosis）が疑われる。鑑別のためにはまず血液検査が必要。しかし，その結果のみで判断するわけではなく，結核の診断には他のテストも必要。

Ⅳ. Further Study

1. Group work: Get information about the infectious diseases that are designated to get vaccination routinely (e.g. measles, varicella, hepatitis B, Hib, etc) under the Preventive Vaccination Act, and present it in English.

   Reference
   1) National Institute of Infectious Diseases（国立感染症研究所）
      <https://www.niid.go.jp/niid/images/vaccine/schedule/2016/EN20161001.pdf>
   2) WHO
      <http://www.who.int/topics/infectious_diseases/en/>

2. Group work: Get information about the worldwide incidence of infectious diseases (e.g. Ebola hemorrhagic fever, avian influenza, Zika virus infection, Dengue fever) and present it in English.

   Reference
   1) Ministry of Health, Labour and Welfare（厚生労働省）
      <http://www.mhlw.go.jp/stf/seisakunitsuite/bunya/kenkou_iryou/kenkou/kekkaku-kansenshou/index.html>
   2) WHO
      <http://www.who.int/topics/infectious_diseases/en/>

3. Get more information about infective endocarditis with an article published in *New England Journal of Medicine*. (Note: This article is available to subscribers only.)

   1) Listen to the audio file without looking at the texts at

      < http://www.nejm.org/action/showAudioSummaryPlayer?uri=%2F doi%2Ffull%2F10.1056%2FNEJMcp1206782&doi=10.1056%2FNEJMc p1206782&aid=clinicalpractice

   2) Then, read the text at

      <http://www.nejm.org/doi/full/10.1056/NEJMcp1206782>

A. Risk factors (male-female case ratio, valve diseases, and other diseases)

B. Presentation and diagnosis (less common signs, and the Duke criteria)

C. Treatment (recommendation for different strains of bacteria)

D. Prophylaxis (guidelines)

11. Uterine fibroid

　子宮筋腫（uterine fibroids, leiomyoma of the uterus）は性成熟期婦人の代表的な良性腫瘍（benign tumor）です。Uterine leiomyoma や fibromyoma とも表現されます。悪性化はないとされていますが，特に子宮平滑筋肉腫（uterine leiomyosarcoma）などの悪性疾患（malignant disease）との鑑別に注意が必要です。年齢や症状により治療は個別化されています。治療を要する人はそう多くありませんが，薬物療法には根治性がありません。一方，子宮全摘術（total hysterectomy）は根治術（radical operation）ですが，妊孕性（fertility）を失うことになります。

Pre-reading activities

Do the following exercise before class.

1. **Where is the uterus located?**

   ....

2. **How large is the normal uterus?**

   ....

3. **What are the uterine fibroids?**

   ....

4. **How many people are suffered from uterine fibroids?**

   ....

5. **What are the symptoms of uterine fibroids?**

   ....

I. Reading

Read the following passages and answer the questions that follow them.

Passage 1

Anatomy

The uterus is located in the center of the pelvis and is the size of a hen's egg. The uterus consists of the uterine corpus (body) and the cervix. The corpus, or body of the uterus, consists of an inverted triangular endometrial cavity surrounded by the myometrium and serosa. The portion of the uterus superior to the endometrial cavity is called the uterine fundus. The cervix is the conduit between the endometrial cavity and the vagina.

inverted triangular
逆三角形の
superior to...
…の上方にある

conduit 導管

Etiology and pathogenesis

Uterine fibroids are a common benign disease of the uterus. They are benign connective tissue tumors found in the myometrium. The incidence of fibroids is 30% in women older than 30 years of age, 50% in women older than 50 years of age. On histological examination, fibroids are composed of well-differentiated whorled bundles of smooth muscle cells that resemble normal myometrium. They grow under the influence of epidermal growth factor and sex hormones, including estrogen and progesterone.

differentiated
分化した
whorled 渦巻き状の
bundle 束

Fibroids can be found in the uterine corpus or the cervix, the latter being much less common. As Figure 1 represents, the fibroids in the uterine corpus can be found protruding into the uterine cavity (submucosal), within the uterine wall (intramural), or beneath the uterine serosa (subserosal). Multiple fibroids are found in up to 85% of patients. The number of fibroids varies, as may their size. Uterine fibroids may weigh up to 5 kg or more. A submucosal fibroid, even of large size, may sometimes become pedunculated as a result of the expulsive action of the uterine muscle and protrude from the cervix; this is called myoma delivery. Intravenous leiomyomatosis and

protrude 突き出る

up to... 最大で…まで

weigh の重さになる

expulsive action
娩出作用

disseminated peritoneal leiomyomatosis (DPL) are unusual variants.

variant 変異型

Symptoms and evaluation

Common symptoms of uterine fibroids include hypermenorrhea (menorrhagia), dysmenorrhea, pelvic pressure, bowel and bladder problems. Uterine fibroids may also cause infertility. Pelvic examination and ultrasonography are generally sufficient to find uterine fibroids. MR imaging can be used to rule out uterine sarcoma, adenomyosis, or ovarian tumor.

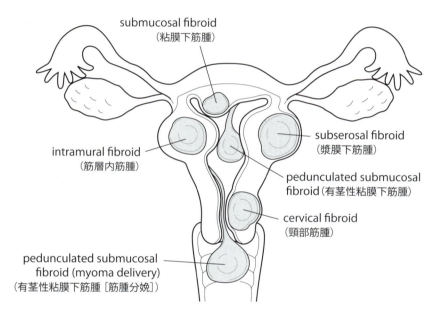

Figure 1. Location and classification of uterine fibroids.

Comprehension questions 1

1. Where can the fibroids be found in the uterine corpus?

2. Which evaluations are generally sufficient to detect uterine fibroids?

Passage 2

Management and therapy

The majority of women with fibroids are asymptomatic. Asymptomatic women should be reassured and followed clinically. For the 30% of women with fibroids who are symptomatic, the choice of management and therapy may depend on symptoms, age, and infertility.

Gonadotropin-releasing hormone agonist (GnRH-a) induces a hypoestrogenic state and therefore can reduce fibroid volume up to 50%; this intervention is done temporarily to prepare for surgery or menopause. Unfortunately, GnRH-a use is limited by its side effects, which include a decrease in bone density.

Surgical myomectomy is the most commonly used treatment for fibroids when future fertility is to be preserved or enhanced. There are a number of different techniques to achieve surgical access for this procedure, depending upon size, number, and location of the fibroids as well as the surgeon's skill and experience. Laparoscopic myomectomy is now widely used; it has advantages over abdominal myomectomy with respect to postoperative pain, duration of hospitalization, and cosmesis. Total simple hysterectomy is also a highly effective treatment for uterine fibroids and other gynecological disorders. Despite advances in laparoscopy, the abdominal route is still more popular than the vaginal, laparoscopically assisted, or total laparoscopic approaches. Laparoscopically assisted vaginal hysterectomy (LAVH) is a type of vaginal surgery assisted by laparoscopic procedures; the success of LAVH depends on the level of difficulty encountered in the vaginal procedure. The vaginal procedure is usually more challenging when the vagina is narrow or uterine mobility is poor. Bleeding in such situations is very stressful for the surgeon. In total laparoscopic hysterectomy

(TLH), all the manipulations except for removal of the uterus are usually conducted laparoscopically. Cases in which application of the vaginal procedure is difficult can be treated with this procedure, but laparoscopic surgery is more difficult.

manipulation 手技

application 適用

Comprehension questions 2

1. How are asymptomatic patients with uterine fibroids managed?

2. Why is the use of GnRH-a limited for patients with uterine fibroids?

3. What are the advantages of laparoscopic surgeries over abdominal surgeries?

4. Why is the abdominal route still more popular in total simple hysterectomy?

II. Vocabulary

☐ abdominal myomectomy	腹式筋腫核出〔術〕
☐ bone density	骨密度
☐ bowel and bladder problems (symptoms)	腸管・膀胱症状
☐ disseminated peritoneal leiomyomatosis (DPL)	腹膜播種性平滑筋腫
☐ dysmenorrhea	月経困難症
☐ endometrial cavity	子宮内膜腔
☐ epidermal growth factor (EGF)	上皮成長因子
☐ estrogen	エストロゲン
☐ fertility	妊孕性
☐ gonadotropin-releasing hormone agonist (GnRH-a)	ゴナドトロピン放出ホルモン作動薬《視床下部ホルモンGnRHの誘導体であり，性腺刺激ホルモン(gonadotropin)の分泌を抑制し，卵巣の機能を抑え，エストロゲンの産生，分泌を抑制する。一時的に閉経と同じ状態にすることで，病巣を小さくする作用がある。》
☐ histological examination	組織学的検査
☐ hypermenorrhea, menorrhagia	過多月経
☐ infertility	不妊
☐ intramural fibroid	筋層内筋腫
☐ intravenous leiomyomatosis	静脈内平滑筋腫
☐ laparoscopic assisted vaginal hysterectomy (LAVH)	腹腔鏡併用下腟式子宮全摘〔術〕
☐ laparoscopic myomectomy	腹腔鏡下筋腫核出〔術〕
☐ menarche	初経
☐ menopause	閉経
☐ myoma delivery	筋腫分娩
☐ myomectomy	筋腫核出〔術〕
☐ myometrium	子宮筋層

☐ ovarian tumor	卵巣腫瘍	
☐ pedunculated submucosal fibroid	有茎性粘膜下筋腫	
☐ pelvic examination	内診《直訳は「骨盤診察」だが，婦人科での「内診」を意味する》	
☐ pelvic pressure	骨盤の圧迫	
☐ progesterone	プロゲステロン	
☐ radical operation	根治術	
☐ salpingitis	卵管炎	
☐ salpingo-oophorectomy	卵管卵巣〔付属器〕摘除〔術〕	
☐ smooth muscle	平滑筋	
☐ submucosal fibroid	粘膜下筋腫	
☐ subserosal fibroid	漿膜下筋腫	
☐ total laparoscopic hysterectomy (TLH)	全腹腔鏡下子宮全摘〔術〕	
☐ total simple hysterectomy	単純子宮全摘〔術〕	
☐ ultrasonography, ultrasound	超音波検査《産婦人科領域では，骨盤(pelvic)超音波検査には，経腹(transabdominal)・経腟(transvaginal)超音波検査が含まれる》	
☐ uterine adenomyosis	子宮腺筋症	
☐ uterine cervix	子宮頸部	
☐ uterine corpus	子宮体部	
☐ uterine fibroid	子宮筋腫	
☐ uterine fundus	子宮底	
☐ uterine mobility	子宮の可動性	
☐ uterine sarcoma	子宮肉腫《子宮体部にできる非上皮性悪性腫瘍。子宮体部悪性腫瘍全体の約8%を占める。肉腫の約半数は癌肉腫(carcinosarcoma)で，残りの大部分を平滑筋肉腫(leiomyosarcoma)，子宮内膜間質肉腫(endometrial stromal sarcoma)，腺肉腫(adenosarcoma)が占める。》	

III. Medical communication

Listen to the recording of the following case report and fill in the blanks. Then do the exercises that follow.

Case report

A ____-year-old woman, gravida ____, para ____, presents with a ____-year history of worsening _____. She reports that during the first several days of her _____ she changes pads (some with _____ _____) every ____ to ____ hours.

On _____ examination, she is noted to have a globular 12-week-size uterus that is freely _____. _____ _____ reveals a uterus measuring over ____ cm with _____ uterine _____. The _____ are normal bilaterally. Figures 2 and 3 reprensent T2-weighted MR images of the patient.

Urinalysis showed no _____. RBC _____ million, Hb _____ g/dL, WBC _____, platelets _____ million, LDH _____ IU, CRP _____ mg/dL, CA125 _____ IU.

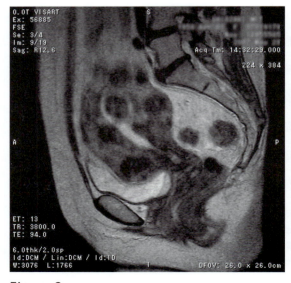

Figure 2.

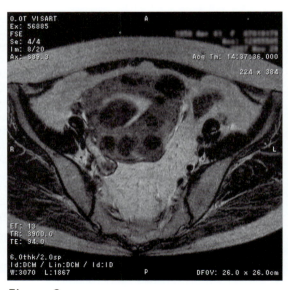

Figure 3.

Clinical exercises

1. **What is the cause of this patient's hypermenorrhea?**

   a   Uterine sarcoma

   b   Adenomyosis

   c   Uterine fibroids

   d   Ovarian tumor

   e   Myoma delivery

2. **What examination will be beneficial to this diagnosis? Choose two.**

   a   Pelvic MRI

   b   Laparoscopy

   c   Abdominal CT

   d   Ultrasonography

   e   Colonofiber

3. **What are possible management for this patients? Choose two.**

   a   Radiation

   b   Estrogen therapy

   c   GnRH-a thrapy

   d   Simple hysterectomy

   e   Salpingo-oophorectomy

Check the answers.

Case report

A **45**-year-old woman, gravida **3**, para **3**,[1] presents with a **2**-year history of worsening **hypermenorrhea**. She reports that during the first several days of her **period** she changes pads (some with **blood clots**) every **1** to **2** hours.

On **pelvic** examination, she is noted to have a globular 12-week-size uterus that is freely **mobile**. **Pelvic ultrasonography** reveals[2] a uterus measuring over **10** cm with **multiple** uterine **tumors**. The **ovaries** are normal bilaterally. Figures 2 and 3 represent[3] T2-weighed MR images of the patient.

Urinalysis showed no **anomaly**. RBC **320** million, Hb **7.8** g/dL, WBC **7,000**, platelets **28** million, LDH **300** IU, CRP **0.1** mg/dL, CA125[4] **25** IU.

gravida 妊娠回数
para 経産回数

period 月経

blood clot 凝血塊

globular 球形の

bilaterally 両側に

T2-weighted MR
image MRI T2強調像
anomaly 異常

Note how the following common terms and phrases are used in case reports.

年齢，性別，主訴と随伴症状について述べる。

❶ A 45-year-old, gravida 3, para 3 female patient presented with …
（45歳，女性。3妊3産。…を主訴に来院した。）

女性患者の場合，年齢や主訴に加え，経妊・経産についても述べる。また，診断をするうえで初経や閉経時期も重要な要素となる。

- A 60 year-old woman with gravida 3, para 2, having had a **miscarriage** at 35 years and **menopause** at 52 years, presented at our hospital for atypical genital bleeding.
  （60歳，3妊2産，35歳時に流産，52歳で閉経した女性。性器出血を主訴に当院受診となった。）

- A 12 year-old **nulligravida** girl, 150.5 cm in height and 45.0 kg in body weight, presented at our department complaining of left lower abdominal pain. **Menarche** occurred at the age of 11 years and 2 months.
  （12歳女児，未妊未産。身長150.5 cm，体重45.0 kg。左下腹部の痛みを訴え，当科受診。初経は11歳2ヵ月。）

❷ A pelvic ultrasound revealed ….（骨盤超音波検査では…が確認された。）

検査所見を述べる際の定型表現。

- Magnetic resonance imaging **showed** a 30×25cm uterine fibroid.
  （MRI検査を行った結果，骨盤内に30×25cmの巨大子宮筋腫を認めた。）

- The results of histological examination **confirmed** uterine adenomyosis.
  （組織学的検査の結果，子宮腺筋症であることが判明した。）

❸ Figures 2 and 3 represent …（図2，3に，…を示す。）

検査所見を図示する際の定型表現。

❹ LDH, CA125

検査所見を述べる際には略語が多用される。（Unit4 Inflammatory bowel disease, P.55参照）

- **LDH**：lactate dehydrogenase（乳酸脱水素酵素；細胞内で糖をエネルギーに変換する際に働く酵素。肝細胞，心筋，骨格筋，血球など全身のあらゆる細胞に含まれており，それらの細胞が障害を受けると血液中のLDHは高値になる。）

- **CA125**：cancer antigen 125（主に卵巣癌に有効な血中腫瘍マーカー。子宮内膜症と子宮筋腫の鑑別にも用いられる。）

11. Uterine fibroid

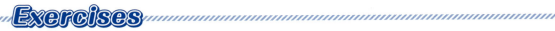

- **Write a case report of the following patient and present it in the class.**

55歳，2妊1産，32歳時に流産，49歳で閉経した女性。腹部膨満感と性器出血を主訴に当院受診となった。内診，経腟超音波検査，MRI検査を行った結果，骨盤内に20×15cmの子宮腫瘍を認めた。腹式単純子宮全摘術，両側付属器摘出術を施行した。手術時出血量は450 mL，子宮重量は1,870 g。組織学的検査の結果，子宮平滑筋肉腫であることが判明した。術後の経過は良好で，術後10日目に退院した。

IV. Further Study

Search for information about the advantages and disadvantages of the surgical treatments of uterine fibroids (including minimally invasive [laparoscopic] surgery and robotic-assisted surgery), along with other methods through the Internet and academic papers. Also briefly explain the obtained information in simple English, the way you would do when talking to a patient.

A. Minimally invasive (laparoscopic) surgery

B. Robotic-assisted surgery

C. Medication

D. Uterine artery embolization (UAE)

E. Focused ultrasound surgery (FUS)

12. Head trauma

　組織や臓器の生理的連続性が破綻することを損傷（injury）と定義しますが，その原因は，創の状態による分類（鋭的，鈍的），外力の種類による分類（高温物質による熱傷，寒冷刺激による凍傷，電気による電撃傷，銃器による銃創，動物・昆虫による咬傷など），受傷状況を加味した分類（墜落・転落，交通，スポーツ，自傷など）のように，多岐にわたります。本章では頭部外傷に焦点を当てます。

Pre-reading activities

Do the following exercise before class.

1. What are the major reasons for the recent increase in the number of patients with traumatic brain injuries?

2. What are the common mechanisms of traumatic brain injuries?

3. What is the major difference in CT findings between subdural hematoma and epidural hematoma?

4. Describe the major mechanism of brain death following head trauma.

I. Reading

Read the following passage and answer the questions that follow it.

In 2013, approximately 2.8 million traumatic brain injury-related emergency department visits, hospitalizations, and deaths (TBI-EDHDs) occurred in the United States. Most of these were TBI-related ED visits (87.9%), and only 2.0% were TBI-related deaths. Males continue to have higher rates of TBI-EDHDs than females. Although the total number of TBI-EDHDs has increased over time, the increases are not uniform across all age groups or principal mechanisms of injury. This suggests that as an area of study TBI-related prevention should be prioritized.

Several hypotheses might explain the increase in TBI-EDHDs over time. First, heightened public awareness about sports-related concussions might have translated into greater public concern about the effects of TBI generally, leading people of all ages to more readily seek care. Second, heightened awareness among health care providers, and the broader dissemination of validated assessment tools, might have resulted in more TBI diagnoses. Although increases were found among youth for TBI-related ED visits, there were also significant increases in the number of ED visits, hospitalizations, and deaths attributable to TBIs among older adults resulting from falls. This across-the-board increase over a relatively short time suggests the need to find ways to prevent and reduce the number of falls resulting in TBI in older adults.

The highest rates of TBI-EDHDs were among the oldest and youngest age groups. TBIs in these age groups are notable for several reasons. In children aged <7 years, TBIs can impair neurologic development and the ability to meet developmental milestones. Impaired development might lead to further challenges as a child ages, such as decline in academic achievement and psychosocial sequelae such as emotional and

concussion 振盪

dissemination
普及，播種

impaired
development
発育障害

sequelae
後遺症，〔二次的な〕結果

behavioral disorders (e.g., depression or attention-deficit hyperactivity disorder). In older adults, TBIs are associated more often with hospitalization and death. As cognitive and physical reserves are diminished at older ages, TBIs might have a greater impact on activities of daily living. TBIs in older adults are more likely to lead to hospitalization, which can be complicated by the presence of comorbidities. Furthermore, more frequent use of anticoagulants among older adults can result in a greater likelihood of secondary effects because of an increased likelihood of intracranial hemorrhage.

The most common principal mechanisms of injury for TBI-EDHDs were falls, being struck by or against an object, and motor-vehicle collisions. Although these three principal mechanisms accounted for approximately 70% of all TBI-EDHDs, particular age groups were disproportionately affected by specific principal mechanisms, as found in previous studies. Approximately half of all fall-related TBI-EDHDs occurred among those aged 0–4 years and ≥75 years. Codes defining whether a TBI was fall-related are heterogeneous. In addition to falls attributable to tripping and slipping, the codes also capture falls on stairs or from ladders, falls from one level to another (e.g., from a bed or a chair), and falls into openings such as swimming pools. This analysis did not examine the individual contribution of each fall-related code. Future analyses should examine these individual codes to better delineate how activities leading to fall-related TBIs vary by age group.

(Adapted from https://www.cdc.gov)

attention-deficit hyperactivity disorder (ADHD) 注意欠陥多動性障害

comorbidity 共存症

anticoagulant 抗〔血液〕凝固薬

intracranial hemorrhage 頭蓋内出血

heterogeneous 同一単位で計れない, 不均質の

delineate 明確にする

Comprehension questions

1. In approximately how many people do TBI-related deaths occur?

2. What is the second hypothesis that results in more TBI diagnoses?

3. In children aged 6 years and younger, what are the effects of TBI?

4. In older adults, what is the likely consequence of TBI?

5. Describe the three most common principal mechanisms of injury for TBI-EDHDs.

Ⅱ. Vocabulary

□ abrasion	挫傷・表皮剥脱
□ assault	〔他人への〕攻撃・傷害
□ autopsy finding	解剖所見
□ Battle's sign	バトル徴候《耳介後部の皮下出血斑で，側頭骨の頭蓋底骨折を示唆する所見》
□ black eye	ブラック・アイ《眼周囲の皮下出血で前頭蓋底の骨折を示唆する所見》
□ brain concussion	脳振盪
□ brain death	脳死
□ brain herniation	脳ヘルニア
□ brain swelling	脳腫脹
□ cardiopulmonary arrest (CPA)	心肺停止状態
□ cardiopulmonary resuscitation (CPR)	心肺蘇生術
□ cerebral contusion	脳挫傷
□ clinical-pathological conference (CPC)	臨床病理カンファレンス
□ coroner, medical examiner	死体検案医
□ death certificate	死亡診断書，死体検案書
□ diffuse axonal injury	びまん性軸索損傷
□ disturbance of consciousness	意識障害
□ epidural hematoma	硬膜外血腫
□ fall, falling	転倒，転落
□ forensic autopsy	法医解剖
□ Glasgow Coma Scale (GCS) □ Japan Coma Scale (JCS)	グラスゴー・コーマ・スケール ジャパン・コーマ・スケール 《いずれも意識レベルの指標》
□ head trauma	頭部外傷
□ hemiplegia	片麻痺

12. Head trauma 163

☐ homicide	他殺
☐ intracranial pressure	頭蓋内圧
☐ laceration	挫創
☐ loss of consciousness (LOC)	意識消失
☐ lucid interval	意識清明期
☐ medical record	診療録
☐ skull base fracture	頭蓋底骨折
☐ skull vault fracture	頭蓋冠骨折
☐ subdural hematoma	硬膜下血腫
☐ suicide	自殺
☐ traumatic intracerebral hematoma	外傷性脳内血腫
☐ vegetative state	植物状態
☐ vehicle collision	自動車事故

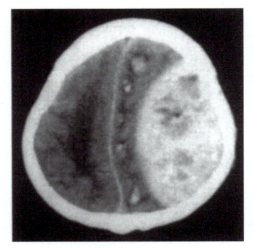 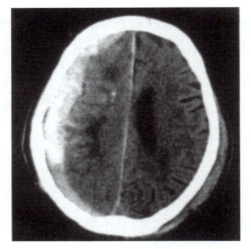

Figure 1. CT images of acute epidural hematoma (left) and acute subdural hematoma (right).

Clinical exercises

When an external force is applied to the head, intracranial changes may occur. Define the major findings listed below:

1. **Subdural hematoma (SDH)**

2. **Epidural hematoma (EDH)**

3. **Cerebral contusion**

III. Medical communication

Listen to the recording of the following case report and fill in the blanks. Then do the exercises that follow.

Doctor-doctor conversation

RP : resident physician   SP : supervising physician

RP : Here is a call from an EMS staff member. A 67-year-old woman who lives with her husband and has a history of _____ heart disease was found lying on the ground near the stairs. Blood was seen on her head. We will have a patient coming in soon with suspected head _____.

SP : Vehicle collision? _____?

RP : Not known.

SP : _____?

RP : On the scene, the woman was drowsy and not responding to _____ commands. Blood pressure of 90/60 mmHg, _____ rate of 110/min.

SP : OK, on arrival, see the patient and run through the case.

The ambulance arrives.

RP : We have a patient here with head injuries. There is a _____ on the _____. Could you come and have a look?

SP : Before that, take vital signs.

RP : Yes, BP 88 over 60, pulse 110. Respiratory rate 28 and temperature of 37.5°C.

SP : Take a drip line. Are you OK? Apply a _____ around the arm 10 cm above the elbow, select a vein, cleanse with alcohol, and insert the needle rapidly and smoothly through the skin into the vein. When blood appears, attach the _____ to the tubing.

RP : Yes.

SP : We need to do a couple of tests. The first one is a CT. Call the _____ staff. Remove all metal or plastic objects, earrings, dentures, and glasses. While we are waiting for the result, contact the next of kin.

RP : Yes.

166

SP : The CT findings revealed _____ hemorrhage and cerebral _____ in the frontal lobe. Typical case!

RP : In what way typical?

SP : The woman suffered an occipital head injury and contusion in the frontal lobe, a so-called contrecoup injury.

RP : I have never worked in the Emergency Room before. Is there any advice you could give me?

SP : Sure. Don't panic, keep cool!

Clinical exercises

1. **What is the cause of this patient's injury?**

   a Assault

   b Heart attack

   c Vehicle collision

   d None of the above

2. **What kind of examination was first performed for the patient?**

   a CT

   b blood test

   c interventional radiology

   d MRI

3. **Which of the following injuries were observed for this patient?**

   a cerebral contusion in the occipital lobe

   b EDH

   c SDH

   d skull fracture

Check your answers.

Doctor-doctor conversation

RP : Here is a call from an EMS staff member. A 67-year-old woman who lives with her husband and has a history of ischemic heart disease[1] was found lying on the ground near the stairs. Blood was seen on her head.[2] We will have a patient coming in soon with suspected head injuries.

SP : Vehicle collision? Assault?

RP : Not known.

SP : Stabilized?[3]

RP : On the scene, the woman was drowsy and not responding to verbal commands.[4] Blood pressure of 90/60 mmHg, pulse rate of 110/min.

SP : OK, on arrival, see the patient and run through the case.

The ambulance arrives.

RP : We have a patient here with head injuries. There is a laceration on the occiput. Could you come and have a look?

SP : Before that, take vital signs.[5]

RP : Yes, BP 88 over 60, pulse 110. Respiratory rate 28 and temperature of 37.5°C.

SP : Take a drip line. Are you OK? Apply a tourniquet around the arm 10 cm above the elbow, select a vein, cleanse with alcohol, and insert the needle rapidly and smoothly through the skin into the vein.[6] When blood appears, attach the catheter to the tubing.

RP : Yes.

EMS: emergency
medical service
救急医療サービス

ischemic heart
disease
虚血性心疾患

occiput 後頭〔部〕

tourniquet 止血帯

SP : We need to do a couple of tests. The first one is a CT. Call the **radiology** staff. Remove all metal or plastic objects, earrings, dentures, and glasses. While we are waiting for the result, contact the next of kin.

RP : Yes.

SP : The CT findings revealed **subdural** hemorrhage[7] and cerebral **contusion** in the frontal lobe. Typical case!

RP : In what way typical?

SP : The woman suffered an occipital head injury and contusion in the frontal lobe, a so-called contrecoup injury.

RP : I have never worked in the Emergency Room before. Is there any advice you could give me?

SP : Sure. Don't panic, keep cool!

subdural
hemorrhage
硬膜下血腫

contrecoup injury
対側衝撃損傷

Note how the following common terms and phrases are used in case reports.

・最初に患者の病歴を明確にする。

❶ A 67-year-old woman has **a history of** ischemic heart disease.
（67歳女性，虚血性心疾患の病歴あり。）

・出血個所から患者の状況を把握する。

❷ Blood was seen **on** her head.（頭部に出血あり。）

・搬送された際の患者の状況。

❸ Stabilized?（安定していますか。）

❹ The woman was drowsy and **not responding to verbal commands**.
（女性は傾眠状態で言葉による指示に反応しなかった。）

❺ Take vital signs.（バイタルをとりなさい。）

❻ Insert the needle rapidly and smoothly **through the skin into the vein**.
（針を速やかになめらかに静脈に穿刺しなさい。）

❼ The CT **findings revealed** subdural hemorrhage.
（CTによって硬膜下血腫が明らかになった。）

12. Head trauma　169

Clinical exercises

Unfortunately, the female patient metioned above has passed away and was autopsied. This case was reported and discussed at the clinicopathological conferece (CPC) as below.

A 67-year-old woman was transported to the ER. She had been found lying on the ground next to the stairs. On admission, a laceration was found on the occipital part of the head and a bruise was noted on the hip. The irregular laceration on the head was associated with a moderately prominent abrasion at the margins. This suggests impact with a flat surface, such as the ground. She began to suffer progressive deterioration over the next few hours. Despite conservative treatment, the woman was pronounced dead on the day after admission.

1. What kind of further injuries are anticipated?

The CT findings on admission showed left anterior subdural hematoma characterized by an area of increased radiodensity with compression of the frontal lobe. Subarachnoid hemorrhage and contusion of the bilateral frontal lobes were demonstrated. In the occipital bone, a skull fracture was also observed. Forensic autopsy was performed 12 hours after her death. Externally, laceration of the occipital head and bruising on the hip were observed. Skull fracture was apparent on the occipital bone which initiated at the site corresponding to the laceration to the foramen magnum. Internally, 20 mL of hematomas were accumulated in both subdural spaces. The brain showed subarachnoid hemorrhage and extensive cortical contusions most dominant in the frontal lobe. Contusions were also seen on the anterior aspect of the bilateral temporal lobes. Cross sections of the brain showed multiple foci of contusion injuries in the cortex of the frontal and lateral lobes. No traumatic changes were found in the neck and chest. At the lumbar region, right iliac bone fracture accompanied by retroperitoneal hemorrhage was found.

2. Describe the contrecoup injury in this woman.

Toxicologically, neither alcohol nor other drugs were detected. The microscopic view of the brain showed areas of extravasation of red blood cells and edematous appearance of the tissues, suggesting an acute change of brain contusion. Finally the woman was diagnosed as dying from head trauma caused by impact to the occipital side of the head.

3. What do you consider the mechanisms of the woman's injuries to be?

IV. Further Study

Search for information about the following terms through the Internet and academic papers. Also briefly explain the obtained information in simple English, the way you would do when talking to a patient.

A. Whiplash injury

B. Diffuse axonal injury (DAI)

C. Shaken baby syndrome

D. Blow-out fracture

Index

A

☐ abdominal distention　腹部膨満感　　64

☐ abdominal myomectomy　腹式筋腫核出〔術〕150

☐ abdominal route　腹式手術　　148

☐ abrasion　挫傷・表皮剥脱　　163

☐ acquired immunodeficiency (immune deficiency) syndrome (AIDS)　後天性免疫不全症候群, エイズ 133

☐ acute appendicitis　急性虫垂炎　　50

☐ acute coronary syndrome　急性冠症候群　　36

☐ acute encephalopathy　急性脳症　　22

☐ acute gastroenteritis　急性胃腸炎　　50

☐ acute kidney injury　急性腎障害　　107

☐ acute metabolic encephalopathy
　　急性代謝性脳症　　22

☐ acute myocardial infarction　急性心筋梗塞　　36

☐ acute poliomyelitis　急性灰白髄炎　　133

☐ acute thrombectomy　急性期血栓除去療法　　8

☐ adult T cell leukemia-lymphoma
　　成人T細胞性白血病/リンパ腫　　121

☐ albuminuria　アルブミン尿　　107

☐ alcoholic liver cirrhosis　アルコール性肝硬変　64

☐ alert and awake　〔意識が〕清明である　　124

☐ α-glucosidase inhibitor
　　αグルコシダーゼ阻害薬　　96

☐ ammonia smell　アンモニア臭　　70

☐ amputation　切断　　93

☐ analgesic　鎮痛薬　　34

☐ aneurysm　動脈瘤　　8

☐ angina [pectoris]　狭心症　　36

☐ angiography　血管撮影〔法〕　　8

☐ angiotensin receptor blocker
　　アンジオテンシン受容体遮断薬　　12

☐ angiotensin receptor blocker (ARB)
　　アンジオテンシン受容体拮抗薬　　107

☐ angiotensin-converting enzyme (ACE) inhibitor　アンジオテンシン変換酵素阻害薬　107

☐ ankylosing spondylitis　強直性脊椎炎　　80

☐ anomaly　異常　　154

☐ anti-arrhythmic agent　抗不整脈薬　　36

☐ anti-coagulant (drug)　抗凝固薬　　8, 161

☐ anti-epileptic　抗てんかん薬　　22

☐ anti-inflammatory drug　抗炎症薬　　84

☐ anti-nuclear antibody (ANA)　抗核抗体　　80

☐ anti-platelet agent (drug)　抗血小板薬　　8, 36

☐ aortic aneurysm　大動脈瘤　　36

☐ aortic regurgitation　大動脈弁逆流〔症〕　　36

☐ arrhythmia　不整脈　　36

☐ arthritis　関節炎　　80

☐ aspirin　アスピリン　　36

☐ assault　〔他人への〕攻撃・傷害　　163

☐ atheroma　粥腫　　36

☐ atherosclerosis　動脈硬化〔症〕　　8

☐ atherosclerotic lesion
　　アテローム（粥状）硬化性病変　　32

☐ atherosclerotic plaque
　　アテローム性動脈硬化性プラーク　　8

☐ athlete's foot　水虫　　135

☐ atrial fibrillation　心房細動　　8, 36

☐ atrio-ventricular block　房室ブロック　　36

☐ attention-deficit hyperactivity disorder (ADHD)　注意欠陥多動性障害　　161

☐ autoimmune hepatitis　自己免疫性肝炎　　64

☐ autologous peripheral blood stem cell transplantation　自家末梢血幹細胞移植　121

☐ autologous stem cell transplantation
　　自家幹細胞移植　　118

☐ automatism　自動症　　22

☐ autopsy finding　解剖所見　　163

B

☐ B symptoms　B症状　　120

☐ bacteremia　菌血症　　133

☐ Battle's sign　バトル徴候　　163

☐ Behçet's disease　ベーチェット病　　80

☐ birth defect　先天性欠損　　22

☐ black eye　ブラック・アイ　　163

☐ blood clot　凝血塊　　154

☐ blood clotting deficiency　血液凝固因子欠乏　5

Index　173

□ blood concentration　血中濃度　　26
□ blurred vision　かすみ目　　91
□ bone density　骨密度　　150
□ bone marrow biopsy　骨髄生検　　120
□ bowel and bladder problems (symptoms)
　　腸管・膀胱症状　　150
□ brain abscess　脳膿瘍　　22
□ brain attack　脳発作　　2
□ brain concussion　脳振盪　　163
□ brain death　脳死　　163
□ brain herniation　脳ヘルニア　　163
□ brain swelling　脳腫脹　　163
□ bronchial asthma　気管支喘息　　26
□ Burkitt lymphoma　バーキットリンパ腫　　121
□ butterfly rash　蝶形紅斑　　80

C

□ C peptide immunoreactivity (CPR)
　　Cペプチド免疫活性　　94
□ C-reactive protein　C反応性蛋白　　32
□ cardiac failure　心不全　　36
□ cardiac sudden death　心臓突然死　　36
□ cardiac tamponade　心タンポナーデ　　36, 116
□ cardiogenic shock　心原性ショック　　36
□ cardiomyopathy　心筋症　　36
□ cardiopulmonary arrest (CPA)　心肺停止状態 163
□ cardiopulmonary resuscitation (CPR)
　　心肺蘇生術　　163
□ cardiotonic agent　強心薬　　36
□ cardiovascular disease　心血管疾患　　36
□ casual plasma (blood) glucose　随時血糖　　94
□ catheter intervention　カテーテル治療　　36
□ catheter-related blood stream infection
　　カテーテル関連血流感染症　　133
□ cellulitis　蜂窩織炎　　133
□ cephalosporin　セファロスポリン系抗菌薬　　133
□ cerebral contusion　脳挫傷　　163
□ cerebral hemorrhage　脳出血　　69
□ cerebral infarction　脳梗塞　　8
□ cerebral thrombosis　脳血栓症　　8
□ cerebrovascular disease　脳血管障害　　8
□ chickenpox　水痘　　135

□ chief complaint　主訴　　69
□ Child-Pugh score　チャイルド・ピュースコア　　63
□ cholangitis　胆管炎　　50
□ cholecystitis　胆嚢炎　　50
□ cholelithiasis　胆石症　　50
□ cholera　コレラ　　133
□ cholestasis　胆汁うっ滞　　60
□ cholestatic cirrhosis　胆汁うっ滞性肝硬変　　64
□ chromosomal abnormality　染色体異常　　116
□ chronic hepatitis　慢性肝炎　　64
□ chronic kidney disease (CKD)　慢性腎臓病　107
□ chronic liver disease　慢性肝疾患　　64
□ chronic lymphocytic leukemia/small
　　lymphocytic lymphoma
　　慢性リンパ性白血病/小リンパ球性リンパ腫　　121
□ Churg-Strauss syndrome
　　チャーグ・ストラウス症候群　　80
□ cirrhosis [of the liver]　肝硬変　　64
□ clinical-pathological conference (CPC)
　　臨床病理カンファレンス　　163
□ clipping　クリッピング術　　8
□ coil embolization　コイル塞栓術　　8
□ colectomy　結腸切除術　　49, 50
□ colon cancer　大腸癌　　50
□ coma　昏睡状態　　22
□ community-acquired infection　市中感染症 133
□ comorbidity　共存症　　161
□ compensated cirrhosis　代償性肝硬変　　64
□ complication　合併症　　34
□ comprehensive physical examination
　　総合的健康診断, 人間ドック　　69
□ computed tomography, computerized axial
　　tomography, CAT scan
　　コンピュータ連動断層撮影〔法〕, CTスキャン　　8
□ concussion　振盪　　160
□ congestive cirrhosis　うっ血性肝硬変　　64
□ congestive heart failure　うっ血性心不全　　131
□ conjunctiva　眼球結膜　　70
□ conjunctivitis　結膜炎　　133
□ consciousness level　意識レベル　　69
□ continuous EEG video monitoring
　　持続ビデオ脳波モニタリング　　22

- continuous subcutaneous insulin infusion 持続皮下インスリン注入療法　94
- contrast enema　注腸造影　68
- contrecoup injury　対側衝撃損傷　169
- convulsion　痙攣, 発作　22
- convulsive status epilepticus (CSE) 痙攣性てんかん重積状態　22
- coronary angioplasty　冠動脈形成術　36
- coronary artery bypass graft (CABG) 冠動脈バイパス術　36
- coronary stenting　冠動脈ステント留置術　36
- coroner　死体検案医　163
- Crohn's disease　クローン病　50
- cryptogenic cirrhosis　潜在性肝硬変　64
- curative therapy　原因療法, 根治療法　64
- cystitis　膀胱炎　133
- cytogenetics　細胞遺伝学　120

D

- death certificate　死亡診断書, 死体検案書　163
- decompensated cirrhosis　非代償性肝硬変　64
- deep vein thrombosis (DVT)　深部静脈血栓症　36
- definitive diagnosis　確定診断　131
- Dengue fever　デング熱　133
- deterioration　悪化　60
- diabetes insipidus　尿崩症　94
- diabetes mellitus, diabetes　糖尿病　94
- diabetic coma　糖尿病〔性〕昏睡　94
- diabetic foot　糖尿病足病変　94
- diabetic glomerulosclerosis 糖尿病性糸球体硬化症　94
- diabetic ketoacidosis　糖尿病〔性〕ケトアシドーシス　94
- diagnostic and therapeutic procedures 診断治療手技　22
- dialysis　透析　92
- diet therapy　食事療法　94
- differential diagnosis　鑑別診断　131
- diffuse axonal injury　びまん性軸索損傷　163
- diffuse large B cell lymphoma びまん性大細胞型B細胞性リンパ腫　121
- diffusion weighted image (DWI)　拡散強調画像　8
- digital rectal examination　直腸指診　70

- dipeptidyl peptidase IV (DPP-4) inhibitor ジペプチジル・ペプチダーゼIV阻害薬　94
- diphtheria　ジフテリア　133
- disease-modifying anti-rheumatic drug (DMARD)　抗リウマチ薬　80
- disseminated peritoneal leiomyomatosis (DPL)　腹膜播種性平滑筋腫　150
- dissemination　普及, 播種　160
- distress　苦痛　40
- disturbance of consciousness　意識障害　163
- diuretic　利尿薬　36
- duodenal ulcer　十二指腸潰瘍　50
- dyslipidemia　脂質異常症　37
- dysmenorrhea　月経困難症　150
- dyspnea on exertion　労作時呼吸困難　131

E

- edema in the lower extremities　下腿浮腫　70
- electroencephalography (EEG)　脳波検査　22
- embolism; embolus　塞栓症; 塞栓　8
- emergency intensive care　救急・集中治療　22
- encephalitis　脳炎　19
- encephalopathy　脳症　19
- end-stage renal disease (ESRD)　末期腎不全　107
- endometrial cavity　子宮内膜腔　150
- endovascular surgery　血管内治療　8
- enterococcus　腸球菌　133
- eosinophilic granulomatosis with polyangiitis (EGPA)　好酸球性多発血管炎性肉芽腫症　80
- epidemic　流行病, 伝染病, 疫病　133
- epidemic parotitis　流行性耳下腺炎　133
- epidermal growth factor (EGF)　上皮成長因子　150
- epidural hematoma　硬膜外血腫　163
- epigastric varices　腹壁静脈怒張　64
- epilepsy　てんかん　22
- epileptic seizure　てんかん性発作　22
- epileptogenesis　てんかん原性　22
- episode　発作　18
- Epstein-Barr virus (EB virus) エプスタイン・バー(EB)ウイルス　120
- erectile dysfunction　勃起障害　93
- esophageal cancer　食道癌　50

Index　175

☐ esophageal varix　食道静脈瘤　　50
☐ esophagogastric varix　食道・胃静脈瘤　64
☐ estimated GFR (eGFR)　推算糸球体濾過量　107
☐ estrogen　エストロゲン　150
☐ etiology　病因　107, 120
☐ excisional biopsy　摘出生検, 切除生検　117
☐ exercise therapy　運動療法　94
☐ expulsive action　娩出作用　146
☐ extraction　摘出, 抽出　130
☐ extranodal lymphoid tissue　節外性リンパ組織　116

F

☐ factitious disease　虚偽性障害　22
☐ fall, falling　転倒, 転落　163
☐ fasting hyperglycemia　空腹時高血糖　94
☐ fasting plasma (blood) glucose (FPG, FBG)
　　空腹時血糖　94
☐ fatty liver　脂肪肝　64
☐ febrile　熱がある　133
☐ fertility　妊孕性　150
☐ fibrinogen　フィブリノーゲン　32
☐ fibromyalgia　線維筋痛症　80
☐ fibrosis　線維化　64
☐ fibrotic proliferation　線維増生　65
☐ fibrous cap　線維性皮膜　37
☐ fine-needle aspirate　細針吸引生検　117
☐ fistula　瘻孔　50
☐ flapping tremor　羽ばたき振戦　68
☐ flare-up　再発　49
☐ fluid-attenuated inversion recovery (FLAIR)
　　フレアー法　8
☐ follicular lymphoma　濾胞性リンパ腫　121
☐ foodborne disease　食品媒介疾患　133
☐ foreign substance　異物　46
☐ forensic autopsy　法医解剖　163
☐ functional dyspepsia (FD)　機能性消化管障害　50

G

☐ gangrene　壊疽　94
☐ gastric caner　胃癌　50
☐ gastric ulcer　胃潰瘍　50
☐ gastric varix　胃静脈瘤　50

☐ gastroesophageal reflux disease (GERD)
　　胃食道逆流症　50
☐ gastroesophageal varix　胃・食道静脈瘤　64
☐ gastrointestinal hemorrhage　消化管出血　64
☐ gastrointestinal obstruction　胃腸管閉塞　116
☐ general malaise　全身倦怠感　65
☐ generalized peritonitis　汎発性腹膜炎　50
☐ German measles　風疹　134
☐ gestational diabetes　妊娠糖尿病　94
☐ giant cell arteritis　巨細胞性動脈炎　81
☐ Glasgow Coma Scale (GCS)
　　グラスゴー・コーマ・スケール　12, 163
☐ glomerular filtration rate (GFR)
　　糸球体濾過量　107
☐ glomerular nephritis　糸球体腎炎　107
☐ glucagon test　グルカゴン負荷試験　94
☐ glucagon-like peptide 1 (GLP-1)
　　グルカゴン様ペプチド　94
☐ glucose transporter (GLUT)　糖輸送担体　94
☐ glucotoxicity　糖毒性　94
☐ glycolysis system　解糖系　94
☐ glyconeogenesis　糖新生　94
☐ gonadotropin-releasing hormone agonist
　　(GnRH-a)　ゴナドトロピン放出ホルモン作動薬　150
☐ granulomatosis with polyangiitis (GPA)
　　多発血管炎性肉芽腫症　80
☐ gravida　妊娠回数　154
☐ gynecomastia　女性化乳房　64

H

☐ *Haemophilus influenzae* type b (Hib)
　　ヘモフィルス・インフルエンザ菌b型　133
☐ head trauma　頭部外傷　163
☐ healthcare-associated infection
　　医療関連感染症　133
☐ heart failure　心不全　36
☐ hematemesis　吐血　64
☐ hematoma　血腫　12
☐ hemiplegia　片麻痺　163
☐ hemodialysis　血液透析療法　107
☐ hemoglobin A1c (HbA1c)　糖化ヘモグロビン　95
☐ hemorrhoidectomy　痔核切除術　54

☐ Henoch-Schönlein purpura
　　ヘノッホ・シェーンライン紫斑病　　80
☐ hepatic encephalopathy　肝性脳症　64
☐ hepatic failure　肝不全　26, 65
☐ hepatic steatosis　脂肪肝　64
☐ hepatitis　肝炎　64
☐ hepatocellular carcinoma　肝細胞癌　65
☐ hepatocellular necrosis　肝細胞壊死　64
☐ hepatocellular regeneration　肝細胞再生　64
☐ hepatomegaly　肝腫大　120
☐ herpes zoster　帯状疱疹　133
☐ higher brain dysfunction　高次脳機能障害　22
☐ higher brain function　高次脳機能　22
☐ histological examination　組織学的検査　150
☐ Hodgkin lymphoma (HL)　ホジキンリンパ腫　120
☐ homicide　他殺　164
☐ homocysteine　ホモシステイン　32
☐ human immunodeficiency virus (HIV)
　　ヒト免疫不全ウイルス　120
☐ human T-cell leukemia virus 1 (HTLV-1)
　　ヒトT細胞白血病ウイルス　120
☐ hyperglycemia　高血糖　90
☐ hyperkalemia　高カリウム血症　107
☐ hyperlipidemia　高脂血症　8
☐ hypermenorrhea　過多月経　150
☐ hyperosmolar hyperglycemic syndrome
　　(HHS)　高浸透圧高血糖症候群　95
☐ hypersplenism　脾機能亢進症　64
☐ hypoestrogenic state　低エストロゲン状態　148

I

☐ idiopathic cirrhosis　特発性（原因不明の）肝硬変　64
☐ ileus　腸閉塞　50
☐ immune response　免疫反応　46
☐ immunoreactive insulin　免疫反応性インスリン　95
☐ immunosuppressant　免疫抑制薬　80
☐ impaired development　発育障害　160
☐ impaired fasting glycemia (IFG)
　　空腹時血糖異常　95
☐ impaired glucose tolerance　耐糖能異常　69
☐ impaired glucose tolerance (IGT)　耐糖能異常　95
☐ incidence　発生率, 発病率　118

☐ incretin　インクレチン　95
☐ indocyanine green test (ICG)
　　インドシアニングリーン試験　63
☐ infarction　梗塞　131
☐ infectious organism　感染性の細菌　130
☐ infective endocarditis　感染性心内膜炎　37
☐ infertility　不妊　150
☐ inflammatory bowel disease (IBD)
　　炎症性腸疾患　50
☐ inguinal hernia　鼠径ヘルニア　50
☐ insulin analog　インスリンアナログ　95
☐ insulin resistance　インスリン抵抗性　95
☐ insulin therapy　インスリン療法　95
☐ insulin-dependent diabetes mellitus (IDDM)
　　インスリン依存性糖尿病　95
☐ intermittent fever　間欠熱　133
☐ International Prognostic Index (IPI)
　　国際予後指数　121
☐ intracerebral hemorrhage　脳内出血　5
☐ intracranial hemorrhage　頭蓋内出血　161
☐ intracranial pressure　頭蓋内圧　164
☐ intramural fibroid　筋層内筋腫　150
☐ intravenous leiomyomatosis　静脈内平滑筋腫　150
☐ intussusception　腸重積症　50
☐ involvement　浸潤　120
☐ irritable bowel syndrome (IBS)
　　過敏性腸症候群　51
☐ ischemic heart disease　虚血性心疾患　168
☐ ischemic stroke　虚血性脳卒中　2
☐ isolated seizure　孤立発作　18

J, K

☐ Japan Coma Scale (JCS)
　　ジャパン・コーマ・スケール　163
☐ jaundice　黄疸, 黄染　54, 65
☐ joint erosion　関節のびらん　80
☐ joint swelling　関節腫脹　80
☐ joint tenderness　関節圧痛　80
☐ jugular venous distension (JVD)　頸静脈怒張　37
☐ ketoacidosis　ケトアシドーシス　92
☐ ketogenic diet　ケトン食　20
☐ kidney failure　腎不全　107

☐ Kussmaul breathing　クスマウル呼吸　95

L

☐ laceration　挫創　164
☐ lactate dehydrogenase (LDH)　乳酸脱水素酵素　120
☐ laparoscope; laparoscopy　腹腔鏡;腹腔鏡検査法　51
☐ laparoscopic assisted vaginal hysterectomy (LAVH)　腹腔鏡併用下腟式子宮全摘〔術〕　150
☐ laparoscopic myomectomy　腹腔鏡下筋腫核出〔術〕　150
☐ leukocytosis　白血球増加症　134
☐ lipoprotein　リポ蛋白　32
☐ liver atrophy　肝臓の萎縮　64
☐ liver cancer　肝癌　65
☐ liver dysfunction　肝機能障害　65
☐ liver failure　肝不全　65
☐ liver supporting therapy　肝庇護療法　65
☐ living-donor liver transplantation　生体肝移植　65
☐ lockjaw　破傷風　135
☐ loss of consciousness (LOC)　意識消失　164
☐ low-grade fever　微熱　130
☐ lucid interval　意識清明期　164
☐ lumbar puncture　腰椎穿刺　6
☐ lung perfusion scintigraphy　肺血流シンチグラフィ　68
☐ lymph node biopsy　リンパ節生検　120
☐ lymphadenopathy　リンパ節症　120

M

☐ malaise　倦怠感　130
☐ malaria　マラリア　134
☐ manifestation　〔症状の〕発現, 徴候　23, 131
☐ measles　麻疹　134
☐ mechanical thrombectomy　機械的血栓除去術　4
☐ medical checkup　健康診断　105
☐ medical examiner　死体検案医　163
☐ medical record　診療録　164
☐ Medusa's head　メデューサの頭　61
☐ melena　下血, 黒色便　64, 70
☐ menarche　初経　150
☐ menopause　閉経　150
☐ metabolic acidosis　代謝性アシドーシス　107

☐ methicillin-resistant *Staphylococcus aureus* (MRSA)　メチシリン耐性黄色ブドウ球菌　134
☐ microalbuminuria　ミクロアルブミン尿　92
☐ microscopic polyangiitis (MPA)　顕微鏡的多発血管炎　80
☐ Middle East respiratory syndrome (MERS)　中東呼吸器症候群　134
☐ mitral regurgitation　僧帽弁逆流(閉鎖不全)症　37
☐ mixed connective disease (MCTD)　混合性結合組織病　80
☐ mononucleosis　単核細胞症　117
☐ morning stiffness　朝のこわばり　80
☐ morphine　モルヒネ　37
☐ mortality　死亡率　92
☐ motor paralysis　運動麻痺　70
☐ multidisciplinary approach　集学的アプローチ, チーム医療　134
☐ mumps　おたふくかぜ　133
☐ muscle (muscular) guarding　筋性防御　51
☐ myocardial infarction　心筋梗塞　37
☐ myocardial ischemia　心筋虚血　37
☐ myoma delivery　筋腫分娩　150
☐ myomectomy　筋腫核出〔術〕　150
☐ myometrium　子宮筋層　150

N

☐ neovascularization　血管新生　95
☐ nephropathy　腎症　92
☐ neurogenic bladder　神経因性膀胱　95
☐ neurological condition　神経学的状態(疾患)　23
☐ neuropathy　神経障害　92
☐ night sweats　盗汗, 寝汗　120
☐ nitrate　硝酸薬　37
☐ non-alcoholic fatty liver disease (NAFLD)　非アルコール性脂肪性肝疾患　65
☐ non-alcoholic steatohepatitis (NASH)　非アルコール性脂肪性肝炎　65
☐ non-epileptic seizure　非てんかん性発作　23
☐ non-Hodgkin lymphoma (NHL)　非ホジキンリンパ腫　121
☐ non-steroidal anti-inflammatory drug (NSAID)　非ステロイド性抗炎症薬　80, 134

□ nonconvulsive seizure　非痙攣性発作　23

□ nonconvulsive status epilepticus (NCSE)
　非痙攣性てんかん重積状態　23

□ nosocomial infection　院内感染症　134

□ nuchal rigidity　項部硬直　68

□ nutritional and metabolic disorder
　栄養代謝障害　65

□ nutritional therapy　栄養療法　65

□ nystagmus　眼振　26

O

□ opportunistic infection　日和見感染症　134

□ oral glucose tolerance test (OGTT)
　経口ブドウ糖負荷試験　95

□ oral hypoglycemic agent　経口血糖降下薬　95

□ orchitis, orchiditis　睾丸炎　134

□ orthopnea　起座呼吸　68

□ orthostatic hypotension　起立性低血圧　93

□ Osler's node　オスラー結節　134

□ osmotic diuresis　浸透圧利尿　95

□ osteoarthritis (OA)　変形性関節症　80

□ osteoporosis　骨粗鬆症　80

□ otitis media　中耳炎　134

□ ovarian tumor　卵巣腫瘍　151

□ overlap syndrome　オーバーラップ症候群　80

P

□ palmar erythema　手掌紅斑　65

□ palpebral conjunctiva　眼瞼結膜　54, 70

□ pancreatic cancer　膵癌　51

□ pancreatic islet transplantation　膵島移植　95

□ pancreatitis　膵炎　51

□ pandemic　広域に及ぶ感染病の大流行　134

□ papillary muscle rupture　乳頭筋断裂　37

□ para　経産回数　154

□ paresthesia　感覚異常　93

□ pathogen　病原菌, 病原体　130

□ pedunculated submucosal fibroid
　有茎性粘膜下筋腫　151

□ pelvic examination　内診　151

□ pelvic pressure　骨盤の圧迫　151

□ peptic ulcer　消化性潰瘍　51

□ perception disorder　感覚障害　95

□ percutaneous catheter intervention (PCI)
　経皮的冠動脈インターベンション　37

□ peritoneal [irritation] sign　腹膜刺激徴候　51

□ peritoneal dialysis　腹膜透析療法　107

□ pertussis　百日咳　134

□ photosensitivity　光線過敏, 日光過敏　81

□ pigmentation　色素沈着　61, 65

□ plaque　プラーク　2

□ pleuritis　胸膜炎　134

□ polyarteritis nodosa　結節性多発動脈炎　81

□ polymyalgia rheumatica (PMR)
　リウマチ性多発筋痛症　81

□ polymyositis/dermatomyositis (PM/DM)
　多発性筋炎/皮膚筋炎　81

□ polyneuropathy　多発性神経障害　93

□ portal hypertension　門脈圧亢進〔症〕　65

□ portosystemic shunt　門脈ー大循環系短絡　65

□ positron emission tomography (PET)
　陽電子放射断層撮影〔法〕　120

□ post operative pain　術後疼痛　148

□ post-hypoxic and post-ischemic
　encephalopathy　低酸素後・虚血後脳症　23

□ postprandial hyperglycemia　食後高血糖　96

□ precancerous lesion　前癌病変　65

□ prevalence　有病率　23

□ progesterone　プロゲステロン　151

□ prognosis　予後　9, 121

□ progressive disease　進行性疾患　107

□ proliferative diabetic retinopathy (PDR)
　増殖糖尿病網膜症　96

□ prolonged apnea　遷延性無呼吸　19

□ prophylaxis　予防　134

□ propofol　プロポフォール　26

□ proteinuria　蛋白尿　104

□ pseudogout　偽痛風　81

□ pseudolobule　偽小葉　65

□ psoriatic arthritis　乾癬性関節炎　81

□ pyelonephritis　腎盂腎炎　134

R

□ radiation therapy　放射線治療　121

☐ radical operation　根治術　151

☐ Raynaud phenomenon　レイノー現象　81

☐ recurrent attack　再発　26

☐ Reed-Sternberg cell
　　リード・スタンバーグ細胞　121

☐ regenerative nodule　再生結節　65

☐ registration study　登録調査　33

☐ remission　〔病状の〕寛解, 回復　78

☐ renal failure　腎不全　92, 107

☐ renal glycosuria (glucosuria)　腎性糖尿　96

☐ renal replacement therapy　腎代替療法　107

☐ renal transplantation　腎移植　107

☐ repetitive blinking　反復性の瞬目　23

☐ respiratory failure　呼吸不全　116

☐ retinal detachment　網膜剥離　92

☐ retinal photocoagulation therapy
　　網膜光凝固療法　96

☐ retinopathy　網膜症　92

☐ rheumatoid arthritis (RA)　関節リウマチ　81

☐ rheumatoid nodule　リウマチ結節　81

☐ risk factor　危険因子　37

☐ Roth spot　ロス斑　134

☐ rubella　風疹　134

☐ rule out　除外する　19

☐ rupture　破裂, 破綻, 断裂　51

S

☐ salpingitis　卵管炎　151

☐ salpingo-oophorectomy
　　卵管卵巣〔付属器〕摘除〔術〕　151

☐ salvage chemotherapy　救済化学療法　118

☐ sarcoidosis　サルコイドーシス　81

☐ scaling　歯石除去　130

☐ scleroderma/systemic sclerosis (SSc)
　　強皮症/全身性硬化症　81

☐ seizure　発作　23

☐ self-monitoring of blood glucose (SMBG)
　　血糖自己測定　96

☐ sequela　続発症, 後遺症, 〔二次的な〕結果　61, 160

☐ serum creatinine　血清クレアチニン　107

☐ serum lactate dehydrogenase (LDH)
　　血清乳酸脱水素酵素　117

☐ severe acute respiratory syndrome (SARS)
　　重症急性呼吸器症候群　134

☐ shingles　帯状疱疹　133

☐ side effect　〔薬などの〕副作用　23

☐ single photon emission computed
　　tomography (SPECT)　スペクト　9

☐ Sjögren syndrome　シェーグレン症候群　81

☐ skull base fracture　頭蓋底骨折　164

☐ skull vault fracture　頭蓋冠骨折　164

☐ sleep deficit　睡眠不足　23

☐ sodium glucose cotransporter (SGLT)
　　ナトリウム・グルコース共輸送担体　96

☐ soluble interleukin-2 receptor (sIL-2R)
　　可溶性インターロイキン2受容体　120

☐ sore　びらん　51

☐ spectrum　スペクトル　32

☐ spider angioma　クモ状血管腫　65

☐ splenic marginal zone lymphoma
　　脾辺縁帯リンパ腫　121

☐ splenomegaly　脾腫　63, 120

☐ staphylococcus　ブドウ球菌属　134

☐ *Staphylococcus aureus*　黄色ブドウ球菌　134

☐ staring　凝視　23

☐ status epilepticus　てんかん重積状態　23

☐ stem cell transplant　幹細胞移植　121

☐ stenosis　狭窄　32

☐ streptococcus　レンサ球菌属　134

☐ stupor　昏迷　6

☐ subarachnoid hemorrhage (SAH)
　　くも膜下出血　9

☐ subdural hematoma　硬膜下血腫　164

☐ subdural hemorrhage　硬膜下出血　169

☐ submucosal fibroid　粘膜下筋腫　151

☐ subpopulation　部分母集団　46

☐ subserosal fibroid　漿膜下筋腫　151

☐ suicide　自殺　164

☐ sulfonylurea　スルホニル尿素　96

☐ susceptibility　感受性, 感染しやすさ　135

☐ symptomatic epilepsy　症候性てんかん　23

☐ systemic infection, systemic infectious
　　disease　全身感染症　135

☐ systemic lassitude　全身倦怠感　65

□ systemic lupus erythematosus (SLE)
　全身性エリテマトーデス, ループス　81

T

□ Takayasu arteritis　高安動脈炎　81
□ temporal arteritis　側頭動脈炎　81
□ tenderness　圧痛　70
□ tetanus　破傷風　135
□ the Modification of Diet in Renal Disease
　(MDRD)　MDRD式　107
□ thrombolysis, thrombolytic therapy
　血栓溶解療法　9, 35
□ thrombosis; thrombus　血栓症; 血栓　9
□ thymol turbidity test　チモール混濁試験　63
□ tinea pedis　足白癬　135
□ tissue-type plasminogen activator (t-PA, tPA)
　組織プラスミノーゲン・アクチベータ　9
□ tonic-clonic seizure　強直性間代性発作　23
□ total laparoscopic hysterectomy (TLH)
　全腹腔鏡下子宮全摘〔術〕　151
□ total simple hysterectomy
　単純子宮全摘〔術〕　151
□ tourniquet　止血帯　168
□ traction retinal detachment　牽引性網膜剥離　96
□ transesophageal echocardiography
　経食道心エコー　131
□ transient ischemic attack (TIA)
　一過性脳虚血発作　9
□ transient neurological attack (TNA)
　一過性神経発作　23
□ transthoracic echocardiography
　経胸壁心エコー　131
□ traumatic brain injury　外傷性脳損傷　23
□ traumatic intracerebral hematoma
　外傷性脳内血腫　164
□ triglyceride　中性脂肪　32
□ tuberculosis (TB)　結核　135
□ tumor suppressor gene　癌抑制遺伝子　120
□ typhoid fever　腸チフス　135

U

□ ulcer; ulceration; ulcerate
　潰瘍; 潰瘍形成; 潰瘍を起こす, 潰瘍化する　51
□ ulcerative colitis　潰瘍性大腸炎　51
□ ultrasonography, ultrasound　超音波検査　151
□ underlying condition　基礎疾患　23
□ uremia　尿毒症　96
□ urinary glucose　尿糖　96
□ urinary microalubmin　尿中微量アルブミン　96
□ urinary obstruction　尿路閉塞　116
□ urine protein　尿蛋白　105
□ uterine adenomyosis　子宮腺筋症　151
□ uterine fibroid　子宮筋腫　151
□ uterine fundus　子宮底　151
□ uterine mobility　子宮の可動性　151
□ uterine sarcoma　子宮肉腫　151

V

□ vaccination　ワクチン接種, 予防接種　135
□ valve replacement　弁置換〔術〕　37
□ valvular heart disease　心臓弁膜症　37
□ varicella　水痘　135
□ varix　静脈瘤　61
□ vasodilator　血管拡張薬　35
□ vegetation　疣贅　135
□ vegetative state　植物状態　164
□ vehicle collision　自動車事故　164
□ ventricular fibrillation　心室細動　37
□ ventricular free wall rupture
　〔心室〕自由壁破裂　37
□ ventricular septal perforation　心室中隔穿孔　37
□ ventricular tachycardia　心室頻拍　37
□ virus-related liver cirrhosis　ウイルス性肝硬変　65

W, Z

□ Wegener's granulomatosis　ウェゲナー肉芽腫　80
□ white nail, white claw　白色爪　65
□ whooping cough　百日咳　134
□ zinc sulfate turbidity test　硫酸亜鉛混濁試験　63

医学・医療系学生のための
総合医学英語テキスト　Step 2

2017 年 10 月 1 日　　第 1 版第 1 刷発行
2023 年 2 月 20 日　　　　第 5 刷発行

■編　集	日本医学英語教育学会
■発行者	吉田富生
■発行所	株式会社メジカルビュー社

〒 162 - 0845 東京都新宿区市谷本村町 2 - 30
電話　03（5228）2050（代表）
ホームページ http://www.medicalview.co.jp/

営業部　FAX　03（5228）2059
　　　　E-mail　eigyo@medicalview.co.jp

編集部　FAX　03（5228）2062
　　　　E-mail　ed@medicalview.co.jp

■印刷所	図書印刷株式会社

ISBN 978-4-7583-0449-8　C3347

©MEDICAL VIEW, 2017. Printed in Japan

・本書に掲載された著作物の複写・複製・転載・翻訳・データベースへの取り込みおよび送信（送信可能化権を含む）・上映・譲渡に関する許諾権は，（株）メジカルビュー社が保有しています．

・ JCOPY 〈（社）出版者著作権管理機構　委託出版物〉
本書の無断複写は著作権法上での例外を除き禁じられています．複写される場合は，そのつど事前に，（社）出版者著作権管理機構（電話 03-5244-5088，FAX 03-5244-5089，e-mail：info@jcopy.or.jp）の許諾を得てください．

・本書をコピー，スキャン，デジタルデータ化するなどの複製を無許諾で行う行為は，著作権法上での限られた例外（「私的使用のための複製」など）を除き禁じられています．大学，病院，企業などにおいて，研究活動，診察を含み業務上使用する目的で上記の行為を行うことは私的使用には該当せず違法です．また私的使用のためであっても，代行業者等の第三者に依頼して上記の行為を行うことは違法となります．